Clinical
Research

Practice and Prospects

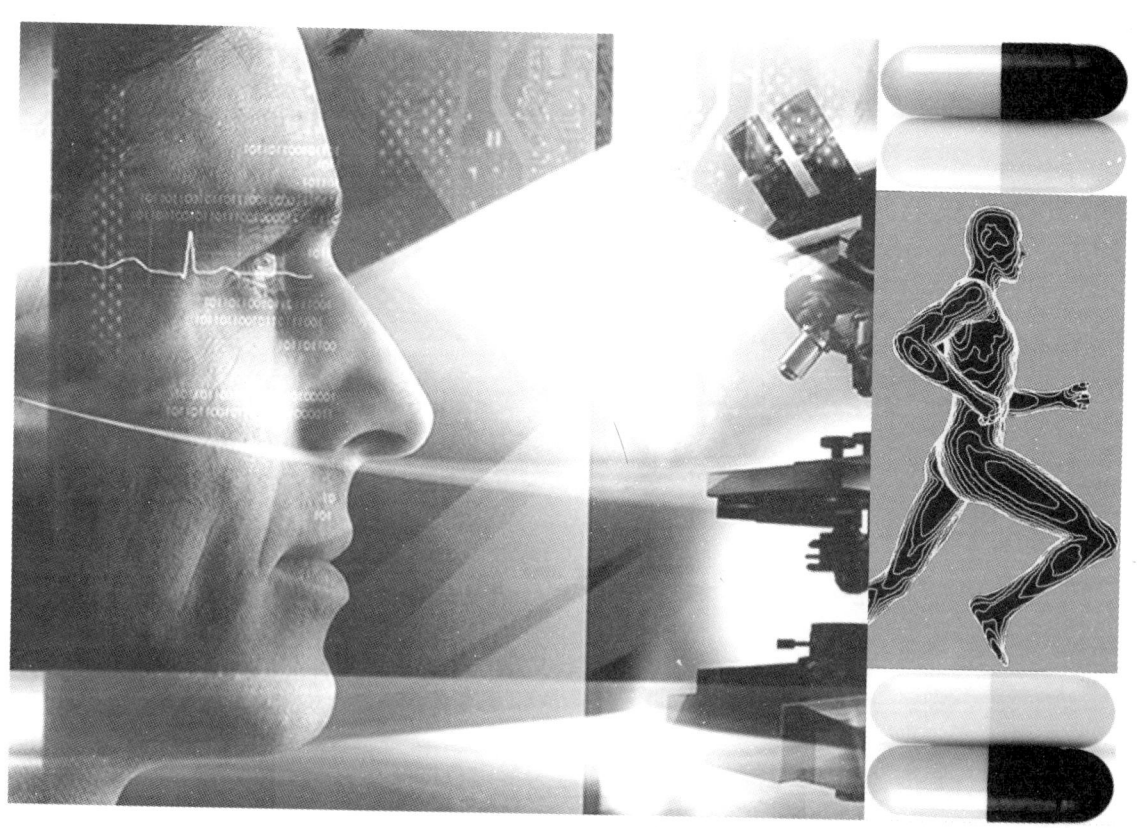

Clinical Research

Practice and Prospects

Editors

T.K. Pal MchE, PhD, VDI (Germany)
Former DAAD Fellow
Director, Bioequivalence Study Centre, and
Head, Department of Pharmaceutical Technology
Jadavpur University, Kolkata

Sangita Agarwal MSc, PhD
Research Scientist
Bioequivalence Study Centre
Department of Pharmaceutical Technology
Jadavpur University, Kolkata

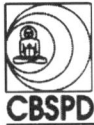

CBSPD

CBS Publishers & Distributors Pvt Ltd

New Delhi • Bengaluru • Chennai • Kochi • Kolkata • Lucknow • Mumbai
Hyderabad • Jharkhand • Nagpur • Patna • Pune • Uttarakhand

ISBN: 978-81-239-1685-9

First Edition: 2009
Reprint: 2014, 2019, 2023

Published by **Satish Kumar Jain** and produced by **Varun Jain** for

CBS Publishers & Distributors Pvt Ltd

4819/XI Prahlad Street, 24 Ansari Road, Daryaganj, New Delhi 110 002, India.
Ph: 011-23289259, 23266861, 23266867
Fax: 011-23243014

Website: www.cbspd.com
e-mail: delhi@cbspd.com;

Corporate Office: 204 FIE, Industrial Area, Patparganj, Delhi 110 092
Ph: 011-4934 4934   Fax: 011-4934 4935

e-mail: publishing@cbspd.com;
publicity@cbspd.com

Branches

- **Bengaluru:** Seema House 2975, 17th Cross, KR Road, Banasankari 2nd Stage, Bengaluru 560 070, Karnataka, India
  Ph: +91-80-26771678/79   Fax: +91-80-26771680   e-mail: bangalore@cbspd.com
- **Chennai:** 7, Subbaraya Street, Shenoy Nagar, Chennai 600 030, Tamil Nadu, India
  Ph: +91-44-26680620, 26681266   Fax: +91-44-42032115   e-mail: chennai@cbspd.com
- **Kochi:** 42/1325, 1326, Power House Road, Opp KSEB, Power House, Ernakulum Kochi 682 018, Kerala, India
  Ph: +91-484-4059061-65,67   Fax: +91-484-4059065   e-mail: kochi@cbspd.com
- **Kolkata:** 147, Hind Ceramics Compound, 1st Floor, Nilgunj Road, Belghoria, Kolkata-700056, West Bengal, India
  Ph: +033-25633055, 033-25633056   e-mail: kolkata@cbspd.com
- **Lucknow:** Basement, Khushnuma Complex, 7 Meerabai Marg (Behind Jawahar Bhawan), Lucknow-226001, UP, India
  Ph: +0522-4000032   e-mail: tiwari.lucknow@cbspd.com
- **Mumbai:** PWD Shed, Gala no 25/26, Ramchandra Bhatt Marg, Next to JJ Hospital Gate no. 2, Opp. Union Bank of India, Noorbaug, Mumbai-400009, Maharashtra, India
  Ph: 022-66661880/89   e-mail: mumbai@cbspd.com

Representatives

• Hyderabad	0-9885175004	• Jharkhand	0-9811541605	• Nagpur	0-9421945513
• Patna	0-9334159340	• Pune	0-9923910676	• Uttarakhand	0-9716462459

Printed at SRK Graphic, Shadara, Delhi

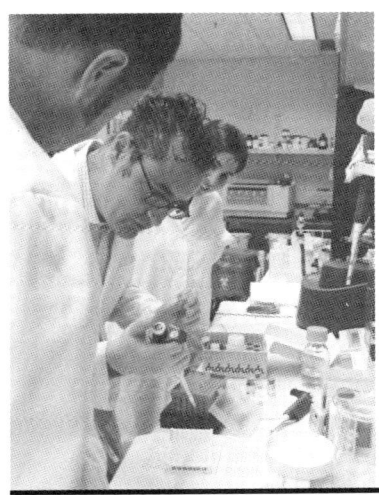

List of Contributors

Anjan Kumar Das MBBS(Cal), MD (Path.)
Assistant Professor
Department of Pathology
CNMC and Hospital, Kolkata 700 014

Arun D Bhatt MD (Med), FICP (Ind)
President, ClinInvent Research Pvt Ltd.
A-302, Everest Chambers
Next to Star TV office, Marol Naka,
Andheri-Kurla Road, Mumbai 400 059

Avijit Hazra MBBS, MD
Lecturer, Department of Dr BC Roy
Postgraduate Institute of Basic Medical
Sciences under (IPGME&R), Kolkata

A. Bose M. Pharm.
Bioequivalence Study Centre
Department of Pharmaceutical Technology
Jadavpur University, Kolkata

B Roy M. Pharm.
Bioequivalence Study Centre
Department of Pharmaceutical Technology
Jadavpur University, Kolkata

CS Deshpande M. Pharm.
Gufic Bioscience Ltd., Mumbai

Gautam Palit MBBS, MD
Deputy Director and Head
Neuropharmacology Unit,
Central Drug Research Institute, Lucknow

Galpalli Niranjan D M. Pharm.
Delhi Institute of Pharmaceutical Sciences and
Research, New Delhi

Kratish Bopanna DSc
Manipal

Krishnangshu Ray
MD (Pharm.), Phd (Med), DA FCCP
Professor of Pharmacology and Medical
Superintendent Cum Vice Principal
RG Kar Medical College, Kolkata

K Veeran Gowda PhD (Pharm.)
Post Doctrol Fellow
Royal College of Surgeons
School of Pharmacy, Ireland

Mita Nandy MBBS, MD (Pharm.)
Vice President
Medical Services and Clinical Research
LG Life Sciences India

Nageshwar Rao Thudi PhD
Group Leader
Bioavaibility and Bioanalytical Studies
Ranbaxy
Canada and USA

N Chatterjee MSc
Bioequivalence Study Centre
Department of Pharmaceutical Technology
Jadavpur University, Kolkata

Parthasarathi Bhattacharyya MD
Institute of Pulmocare and Research, Kolkata

R. N. Sahoo
Gufic Bioscience Ltd., Mumbai

Sangita Agarwal MSc, PhD
Research Scientist, Bioequivalence Study Centre
Department of Pharmaceutical Technology
Jadavpur University, Kolkata

S. S. Agarwal PhD
Delhi Institute of Pharmaceutical Sciences and
Research, New Delhi

S. Shah MD
Nanavati Hospital, Mumbai

S. Darbar MSc
Bioequivalence Study Centre
Department of Pharmaceutical Technology
Jadavpur University, Kolkata

Shawon Lahiri PhD
Central Drug Research Institute
Post Box 173, Lucknow 226001

Suresh K Gupta PhD
Dean, Institute of Clinical Research, India

Tapan Kumar Pal MchE, PhD, VDI (Germany)
Former DAAD Fellow
Director, Bioequivalence Study Centre, and
Head, Department of Pharmaceutical Technology
Jadavpur University, Kolkata

TK Chattaraj MBBS, MD
Clinical Pharmacologist and
Former Associate Professor
NRS Medical College and Hospital, Kolkata

Umakanta Sahoo MBA, PhD
Managing Director
Chiltern International Pvt Ltd., Mumbai

Uttam Kumar Mandal PhD
Department of Pharmaceutical Chemistry,
University of Geneva, Switzerland

Vivek Dhole MSc, PhD
Deputy General Manager and Head,
Application and Training Department
Chemito Technologies Pvt Ltd, Nasik

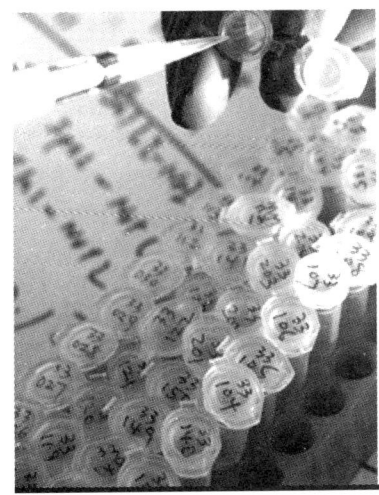

Preface

The Bioequivalence Study Centre (approved by DCGI), the only one of its kind in eastern region at Jadavpur University has been carrying out bioequivalence study of drug molecules for the last six years rendering services to a large number of pharmaceutical industries all over India. Under the guidance and constant encouragement of Prof. A.N. Basu and Prof. S.K. Sanyal, ex-Vice Chancellors, Prof. S. Dutta, Vice-Chancellor, Jadavpur University, and Prof. M.K. Mitra, Dean, FET, Jadavpur University, the University has established a separate full-fledged Bioequivalence Study Centre with the necessary instrumental facilities of global standard. The Centre is thankful to Department of Science and Technology (DST), Government of India, for providing us the LCMS/MS. Special thanks are also due to Dr. G.J. Samathanam, Adviser, Scientist-G, DST, for this kind support in this regard under DPRP programmes.

Presently, Bioequivalence Study Centre in collaboration with International Medical Research Organization (IMRO), Kolkata, and the other medical colleges, has undertaken some of the clinical trials and pharmacodynamic studies using the existing facilities. Compared to the other regions of India, the eastern region has not flourished to that extent in this area. A need was felt, therefore, for both facilities and the expertise existing in the eastern region to undertake clinical trials. Distinguished scientists from various organizations of international repute were, therefore, invited to express their views in this regard. This book contains the papers which were presented at this national seminar which was organized by the Bioequivalence Study Centre.

To conduct clinical studies fairly, it is necessary to understand the concerned principles of research design. With increasing complexities in clinical research, it is imperative that clinical researchers must receive a minimum basic training and awareness in methodology and techniques. Proper expansion of clinical research cannot succeed without the wholehearted support of academia, industry regulators and the civil society. It is vital, therefore, to develop robust mechanisms for cooperation between these stakeholders. The objective of this book is to provide formalized training and awareness in conducting the clinical trials. It is expected that the seminar findings will act as a stimulus to discuss and channelise ideas on various aspects of clinical Research, good clinical practices, ethical issues, data capturing and management, opportunities and challenges, clinical trial monitoring, novel bioanalytical techniques, etc.

The purpose of this book is to assist coordinators, research associates, students and the faculty, and scientists and executives of pharmaceutical industries in creating an awareness about the infrastructure and expertise necessary for conducting clinical research and extend their cooperation in making India a hub for clinical trials with the mission of availing global opportunities.

Realizing the challenges that lie ahead and the huge market potential that is unfolding, this book has been compiled to cater to the needs of the industry. It is sincerely hoped the book will serve the intended purpose and contribute to the development of clinical research of future.

Prof. (Dr) T.K. Pal
Dr. (Mrs) Sangita Agarwal

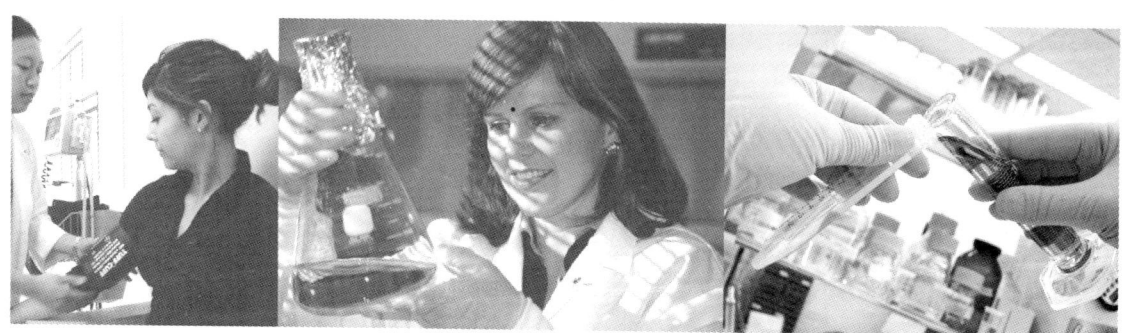

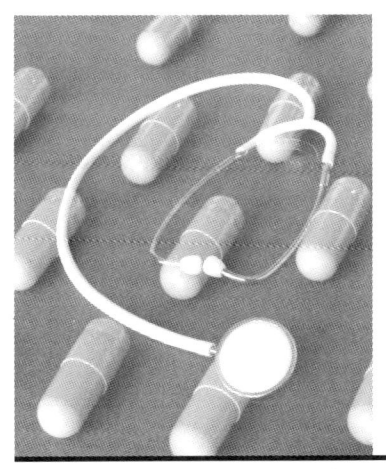

Contents

12. Repeated Dose Subchronic Oral Toxicity Study of Aceclofenac Sodium in Experimental Rats (28 days)

S. Darbar, A. Bose, N. Chatterjee, B. Roy,
U. Mandal, T.K. Chattaraj, T.K. Pal, A. Das

Appendices

Appendix 1   Protocol for Bioequivalence Study

Appendix 2

Appendix 3

Index

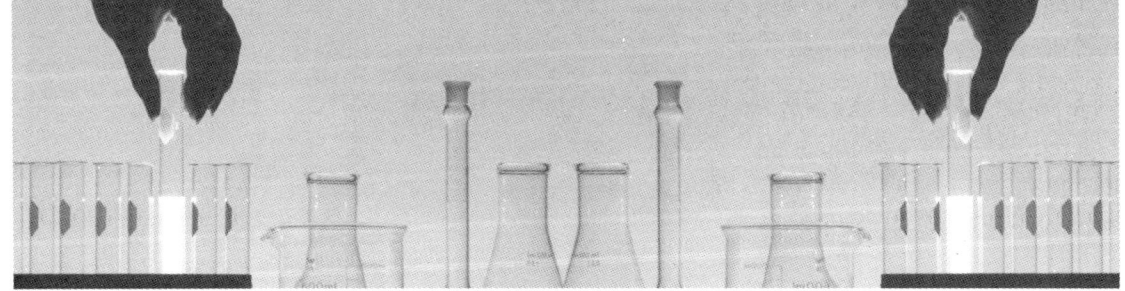

Chapter 1

Clinical Research: From Evolution to Revolution

K. Veeran Gowda
T.K. Pal

INTRODUCTION

India is exploding in the area of clinical research. In the past few years the country has witnessed many multinational companies outsourcing their clinical trial activities to India. This article briefly describes the process of clinical research and its changing scenario in India and worldwide.

History

As per the sources, the first recorded clinical trial was of the biblical Daniel wherein a diet of pulses was tested in humans. But the Royal College of Physicians of Edinburgh, an online resource for clinical trials reports that Daniel's was the first recorded trial, the second was from the 11th century China and the third was from the 16th century France. But the Edinburgh surgeon James Lind (1716–94) who investigated the best treatment for scurvy was the first person to have conducted a controlled clinical trial of the modern era sera[1].

What is a Clinical Trial?

As per the Guidelines of Clinical Practice (GCP) a clinical trial is any investigation in human subjects intended to discover or verify the clinical, pharmacological and/or other pharmacodynamic effects of an investigational product, and/or to identify any adverse reactions to an investigational product, and/or to study absorption, distribution, metabolism and excretion of an investigational product with the object of ascertaining its safety and efficacy. The terms clinical trial and clinical study are synonymous.

Testing in Humans

The process of bringing a new molecule from lab scale to the market is expensive and very tedious. Figure 1.1 explains the whole process of drug development. The success rate of new chemical entity (NCE) development is very low. Only one out of every 10,000 molecules tested reaches the market (Figure 1.2). Before a pharmaceutical company can initiate testing in humans, it must conduct extensive preclinical or laboratory research. This research typically involves years of experiments in animal and human cells. The compounds are also extensively tested in animals. Pharmacology and toxicology studies in preclinical stage are conducted to select or reject lead candidate, indicate the suitability of the drug and for dose selection and guidance to the clinician.

If this stage of testing is successful, a pharmaceutical company provides this data to the Food and Drug Administration (FDA), requesting approval to begin testing the drug in humans. This is called an Investigational New Drug application (IND). The clinical testing of experimental drugs is normally done in three phases, each successive phase involving a larger number of people.

Phase One Study

Phase I studies are primarily concerned with assessing the drug's safety. This initial phase of testing in humans is done in a small number of healthy volunteers (20 to 100). The fate of a drug when administered to the humans is investigated in this phase. The absorption, distribution, metabolism and excretion characters of a drug are studied. The side effects that occur as dosage levels are increased are studied in this phase. This initial phase of testing typically takes several months. About 70 percent of experimental drugs pass this initial phase of testing.

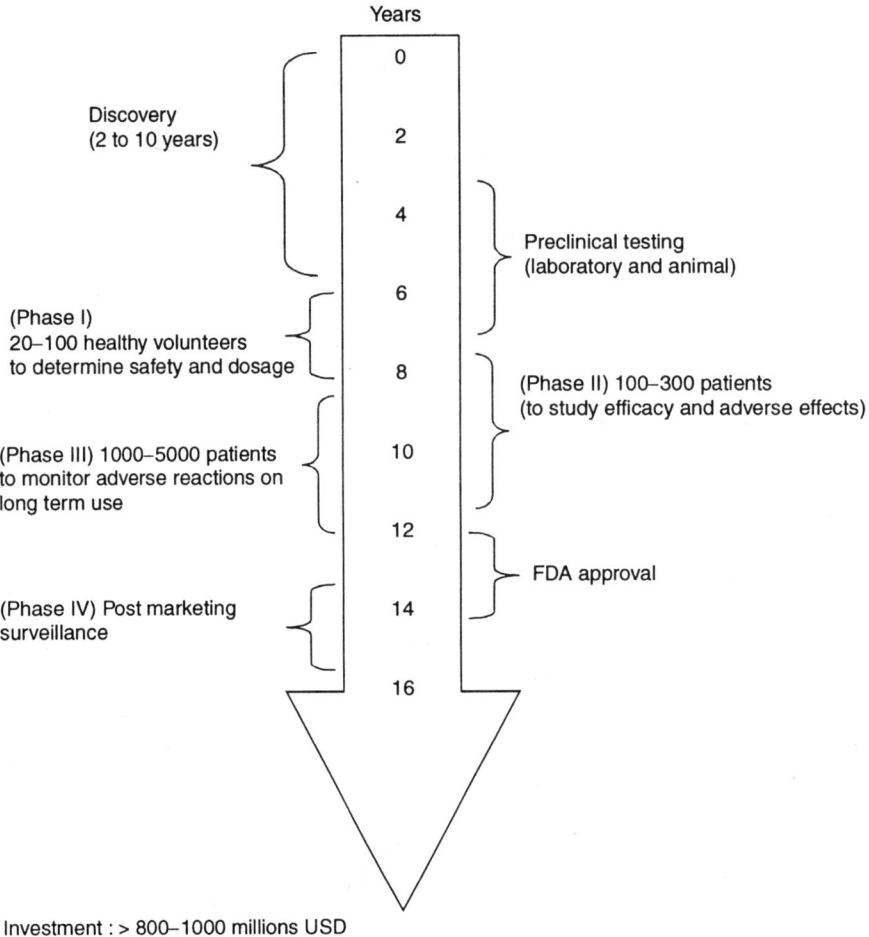

Fig. 1.1. New chemical entity (NCE) development time line

Phase Two Study

Once a drug has been shown to be safe, it must be tested for efficacy. Most phase II studies are randomized trials carried on 100–300 patients. One group of patients will receive the experimental drug, while a second "control" group will receive a standard treatment or placebo. Often these studies are "blinded"—neither the patients nor the researchers know who is getting the experimental drug. In this manner, the study can provide the pharmaceutical company and the FDA comparative information about the relative safety of the new drug, and its effectiveness. Only about one-third of experimental drugs successfully complete both phase I and phase II studies. This second phase of testing may last from several months to two years, and may involve up to several hundred patients.

Phase Three Study

In a phase III study, a drug is tested in several hundred to several thousand patients (1000–3000). This large-scale testing provides the pharmaceutical company and the FDA with a more thorough understanding of the drug's effectiveness, benefits, and the range of possible adverse reactions. Most phase III studies are randomized and blinded trials. Phase III studies typically last several years. Seventy to ninety percent of drugs that enter phase III studies successfully complete this phase of testing. Once a phase III study is successfully completed, a pharmaceutical company can request FDA approval for marketing the drug.

Post-Marketing — Late Phase Three/Phase Four Studies

In late phase III/phase IV studies, pharmaceutical companies have several objectives: (1) these studies often compare a drug with other drugs already in the market; (2) studies are often designed to monitor a drug's long-term effectiveness and impact on a patient's quality of life; and (3) many studies are designed to determine the cost-effectiveness of a drug therapy relative to other traditional and new therapies.

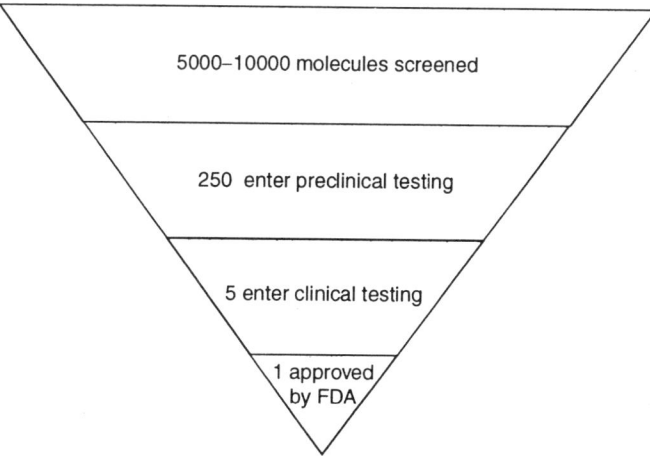

Fig. 1.2. Success rate of new chemical entities (NCEs)

CLINICAL RESEARCH MARKET ANALYSIS

As per the Center watch estimates, the global clinical trials industry is currently worth an estimated $15 billion (Figure 1.3) and has the potential for considerable growth in the future. Global revenues from clinical trials have increased by almost 15% in the last year and the industry is prepared for an extended period of healthy growth. Table 1.1 shows the market share of Indian CROs as compared to Global market.

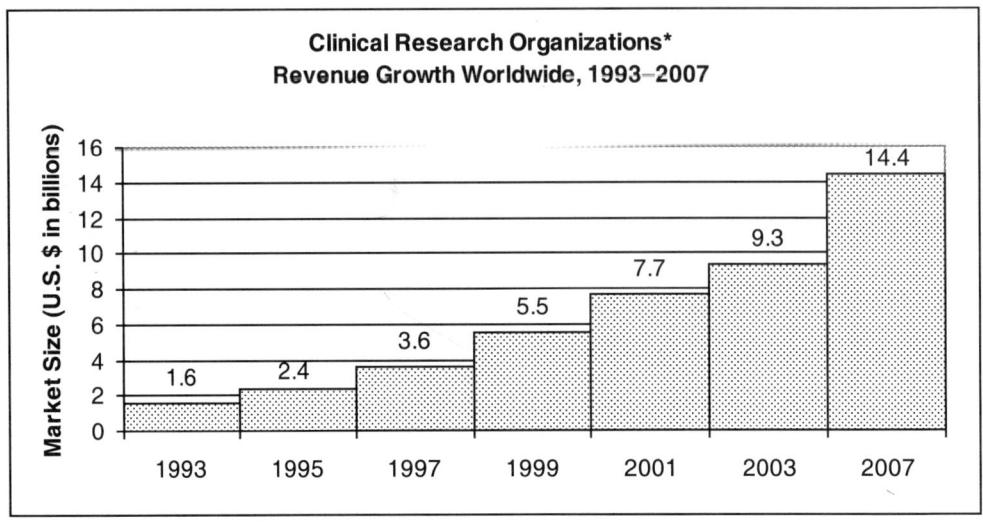

Fig. 1.3. Center watch estimates; World Contract Research Organizations Markets, Frost and Sullivan, 2003

Table 1.1: Survey of Indian and Global Clinical Research Market (McKinsey 2003)

Year	Indian market (Rs. in cr.)	Indian Market (million $) [% of global]	Global Market (million $)
2003	315	70 [1.16 %]	5000–6000
2004	450	100 [1.11 %]	9,000
2005	810	180 [1.80 %]	10,000
2007	2700	600 [2.26% of US]	26,500 US + Rest
2010	4500	1,000 [2 %]	50,000

The Indian pharmaceutical industry is highly fragmented with about 24,000 players (around 330 in the organised sector). In volume terms, it is the world's fourth largest market in unit sales, but ranks 13th in value terms with an annual revenue of approximately 5 billion USD. The top ten companies make up for more than a third of the market. The revenues generated by the industry are approximately US$ 5.2 bn and have grown at an average rate of 8% over last five years. In comparison to the total number of trials done globally, India does just 5–10% of it currently. But this figure is increasing. Companies in the West have realised that about 1/3rd of the urban and urban centric population in India mirror the profiles in the West. The revenues of the top 5 CROs in India crossed 1000 mn in '04 (Table 1.2). Analysis of the CRO market revealed that there are huge number of molecules in Phase II and III stages. Studies involving preclinical testing are also on the rise (Figure 1.4).

According to Center watch, it is estimated that 20–30 percent of global clinical trial activities are being conducted in developing countries. The Indian clinical trials market has grown from $35 million in 2002 to $120 million in 2006. The projected growth by 2010 is $250–300 million. Clinical research can be broadly divided into three areas : hospital site management, database management, and monitoring. Of this, database management constitutes the biggest segment and has the potential to become a $400–600 million business in the next few years.

Table 1.2: Revenues of top 5 Indian CROs, (2003–04), Source: Frost & Sullivan

Company	Revenues (Rs. million)
Quintiles	625.5
Syngene	384.8
Vimta labs	315.1
Pfizer	180
Lambda therapeutics	160
Top 5	**1701.4**
Others	**1050.0**
Total Bio services revenue	**2751.4**

CRO Industry Analysis: 2004 Market (in US billions)

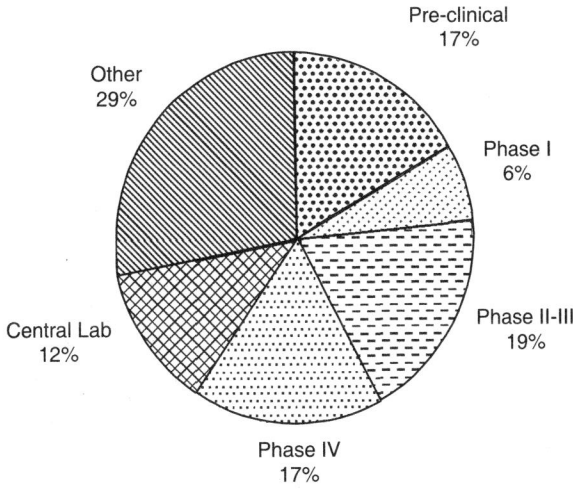

Fig. 1.4. Worldwide CRO market share

Currently there are more than 65 CROs operating in India of which more than 20 are in Bangalore alone. This is mainly because Bangalore has a good network of hospitals, large number of medical colleges, Govt. research institutions and a huge number of IT companies. Some of the leading CROs operating in India are Quintiles, SIRO Clin Pharm, Chiltern, Pharm Olam, iGATE, Acunova, Lotus labs,

Lambda therapeutics, PharmaNet, Synchron labs, Vimta labs, etc. With the much gung-ho on the CRO business, a prevailing trend is the entry of pharma giants like Ranbaxy, Jubilant, Orchid, Torrent, Wockhardt, Sun Pharma and Glenmark in the contract research fray.

Academic Initiatives

The Govt. of India has also been very supportive in this regard to promote research at the academic level. The Department of Science & Technology (DST) has set up 3 National faculties on Bioavailability/bioequivalence studies at CDRI (Lucknow), NIPER (Mohali), Jadavpur University, Kolkata. The centre at Jadavpur University approved by DCGI is also involved in carrying out toxicology studies, clinical trials and other services to the pharmaceutical industries. Over the last few years, the Indian Govt. through its various funding agencies has contributed in organizing workshops, seminars and conferences on clinical research to create more awareness among the scientific community working in academic institutions and the industry.

OUTSOURCING AT A GLANCE

Outsourcing in general means, allowing others do it for you. But the question here is why should others do it for you?

The benefits of outsourcing any job mentioned below might answer this question:

- Cost savings — Definitely, a portion of your cost savings will go to the outsourcer, but outsourcing vendors have a tighter control of fringe benefits and run leaner overhead structures. They also know how to deal with vendors serving the function they are providing and, therefore, are able to pass on to your company the benefits derived from bulk purchasing and effective leasing. By outsourcing a capital intensive function, you can also reduce the costs of equipment obsolescence and depreciation. Costs involved in recruitment, training supervision and other activities can be reduced.
- Quality of service — Because you are doing a certain job for some other company you can develop a "can-do attitude," which may not always be exhibited by an in-house staff.
- More capital funds — Outsourcing reduces the need to invest capital in non-core business functions, thereby freeing capital to invest in other profit-making aspects of the business.
- State-of-the-art technology — Outsourcers have to spend time and money on the most current equipment and on employee training to remain competitive. By outsourcing certain areas, you are assured of receiving the most efficient services and the latest technological advances within that particular function.
- Price stability — By signing a contract to outsource, you will likely be able to obtain stable pricing, eliminating the future need to shop around. Stable pricing allows the company to budget operating expenses and capital purchases more accurately, while potentially preventing the likelihood of surprise expenses.
- New business partners — Outsourcers clearly wish to be viewed as your business partner. And as a business partner, they share in the desire to keep your company operating at its maximum potential. Through this business partner arrangement, outsourcers are eager to introduce you to other outsourcers to assist in that goal.
- More time to focus on core business activities — You cannot overlook this intangible benefit of outsourcing. If a company is to be successful and profitable, management is needed to spend time planning and directing the company's business strategies and not wasting time worrying about managing certain administrative or ancillary function.

Other reasons

- Non-availability of services in-house
- Less knowledge of regulatory affairs in a particular country of interest
- Increased complexity of clinical trials
- Increased amount of data required from clinical trials
- Multinational and multi-center nature of current clinical trials
- Large requirement of patient populations
- Regionalized diseases

Types of Outsourcing Activities

The 2nd Annual Contract Pharma Outsourcing Survey involved more than 200 sponsor-side respondents which involved the various types of outsourcing activities offered and the factors considered while outsourcing any job (Figures 1.5 and 1.6). Analytical testing services followed by API manufacturing and other R&D related activities were outsourced to the maximum. The survey revealed that confidentiality and quality of the data generated were important factors while outsourcing a particular job.

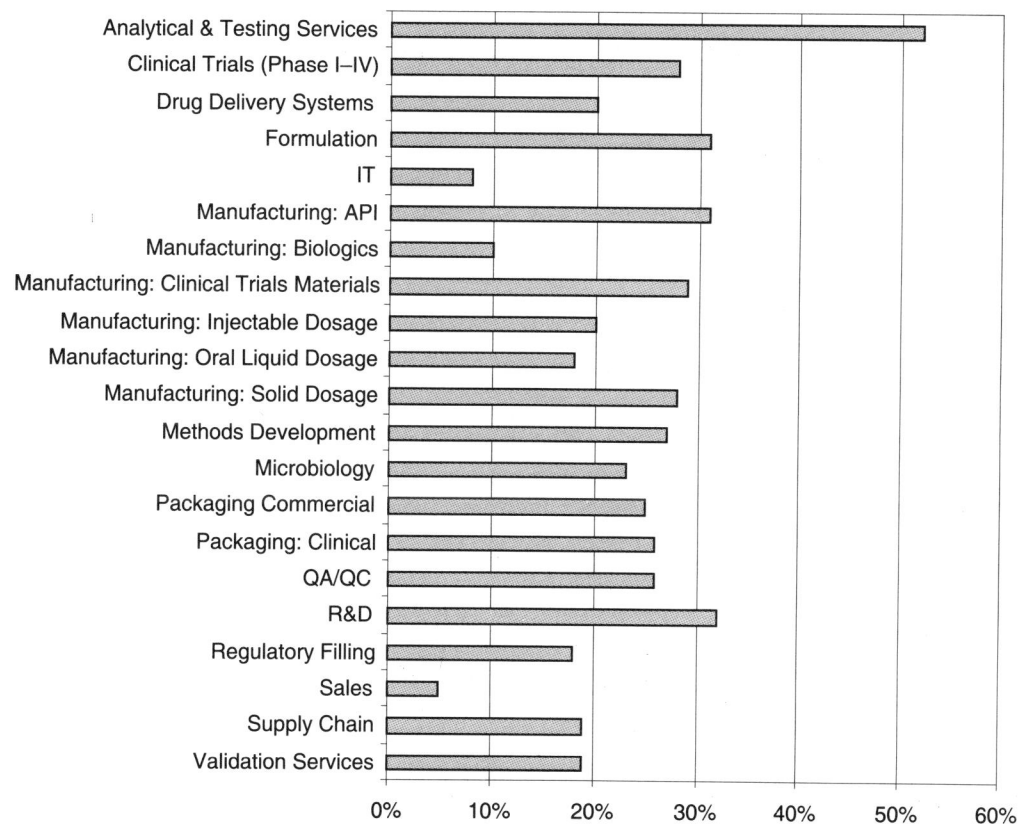

What types of outsourcing decisions are you involved in?

Fig. 1.5. Survey of various types of outsourcing activities

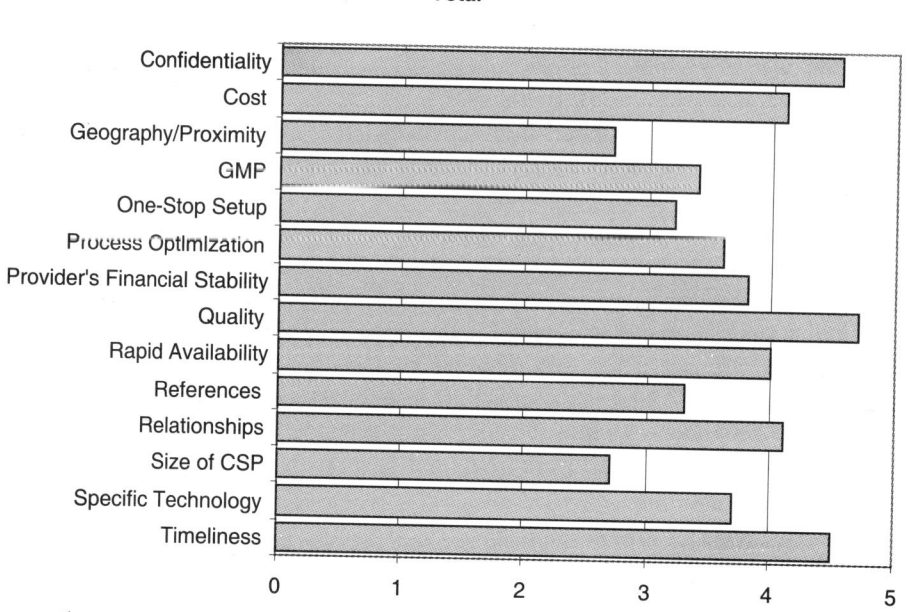

Fig. 1.6. Factors considered by the companies while outsourcing their activities to others

Outsourcing of Clinical Research Activities

To understand why developing countries have become a hot spot for clinical research, one needs to look at the drug development process in totality. This process, which starts in the research labs and ends with a drug being launched in the market, is not only time consuming; it is also extremely expensive. The cost of drug development is estimated at $1 bn, and clinical trials on humans — a critical phase in new drug development accounts for 40% of the total cost.

The main reason for outsourcing is declining productivity of R&D activities (Figure 1.7) and increase in the development time of the new chemical entities. Large pharmaceutical companies like Pfizer have grown mainly because of their outsourcing activities.

The current (2007) estimated market value for R&D outsourcing globally is around 25 bn USD (Figure 1.8) of which the CRO market share alone is 17 bn USD. This promises that Contract Research is going to shoot up like never before in the coming years. In yet another recent global study conducted by consulting firm AT Kearney says that India is the second most preferred destination for outsourcing of clinical trials for the pharma industry. China tops the list and Russia figures as a close third. The study was done across 15 countries and saw India scoring with a large patient pool, faster enrollment and low cost. The study says that the areas that are outsourced include clinical trial data management, data management, parts of IT, payroll, logistics, HR. With maturity of the supply market, functions like stability studies and toxicity evaluation are also being off shored to India.

The study looked at factors like patient availability, cost efficiency, relevant expertise, regulatory conditions and national infrastructure availability. "India scored with its large and relatively naive patient population". This availability helps reduce lead time for patient recruitment by 30–40%. The second advantage is the cost factor. Clinical trials in India, for instance, cost 50% to 60% less than the average cost in the US, says Abhishek Poddar, senior manager, AT Kearney.

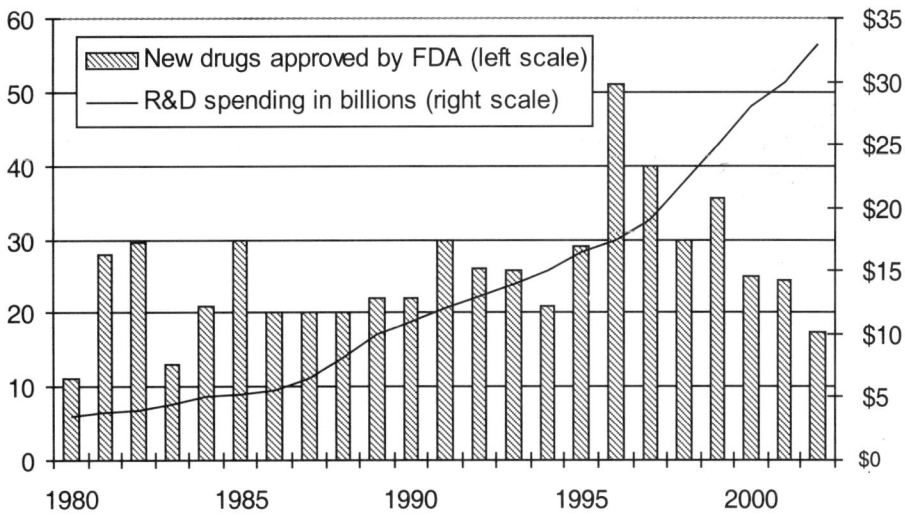

Fig. 1.7. Downfall in the R&D productivity

According to US government publications, today, 8.9% of clinical trials registered with US health authorities are conducted in emerging countries of Asia — 7.4% in Latin America, 7.1% in Central and Eastern Europe and 1.6% in Africa. With 429 clinical trials currently being carried out in the country, Mexico stands out as the most attractive destination for clinical trials outsourcing. Taiwan comes second with 406 trials followed by Poland, Lebanon and Brazil, where 200, 193 and 161 trials are respectively being carried out.

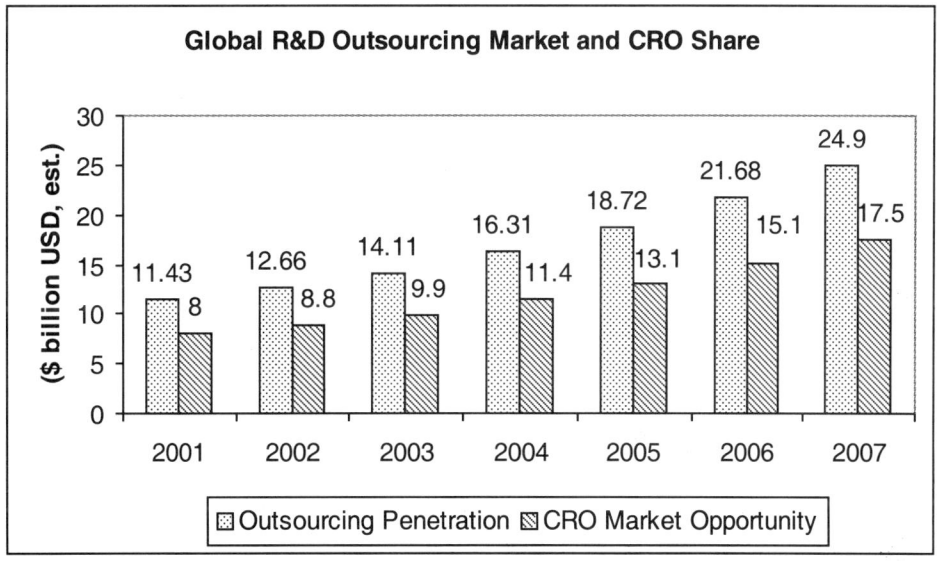

Fig. 1.8. Worldwide R&D outsourcing market

Source: A New Global Outsourcing Market Model to 2007, Goldman Sachs, September 2003.

But more than cost, time is a crucial factor for pharma companies. Considering the fact that a patent lasts 20 years, starting from the moment the drug is discovered and approved for clinical trials, more than half of the time is already gone by the time the trials are over and the drug is finally marketed. Indeed, clinical trials alone can last up to 10 years. And the best way to reduce time is to recruit patients quickly, which is increasingly difficult to achieve in Western countries. India, with large diversity in patient population and disease profiles, is the preferred destination.

Current outsourced clinical trial activity in India is at around Rs. 3.5 billion (about US $ 75 million) and is estimated to go up to Rs. 13.2 billion (about US $ 281 million) by 2010. According to statistics compiled by the Indian Council of Medical Research (ICMR), the total turnover from clinical trials in India in '03 was Rs. 2.25 billion.

A large native patient population pool, various disease profiles and robust infrastructure position India high on the outsourcing list. Today, 122 clinical trials are being conducted in India. GlaxoSmithKline, among the world's top ten global pharma majors, is currently carrying out the largest number of clinical trials in India.

Why India?

Just as the Gulf has its natural resources in crude oil and South Africa in diamonds, India's natural resource lies in its abundant technically skilled manpower (Figure 1.9). India is the world's second largest exporter of software (after the US), and is the source of management and technical talent for over 40 per cent of new start-ups in Silicon Valley. Table 1.3 explains strengths and drawbacks of India as compared to China and other Western countries

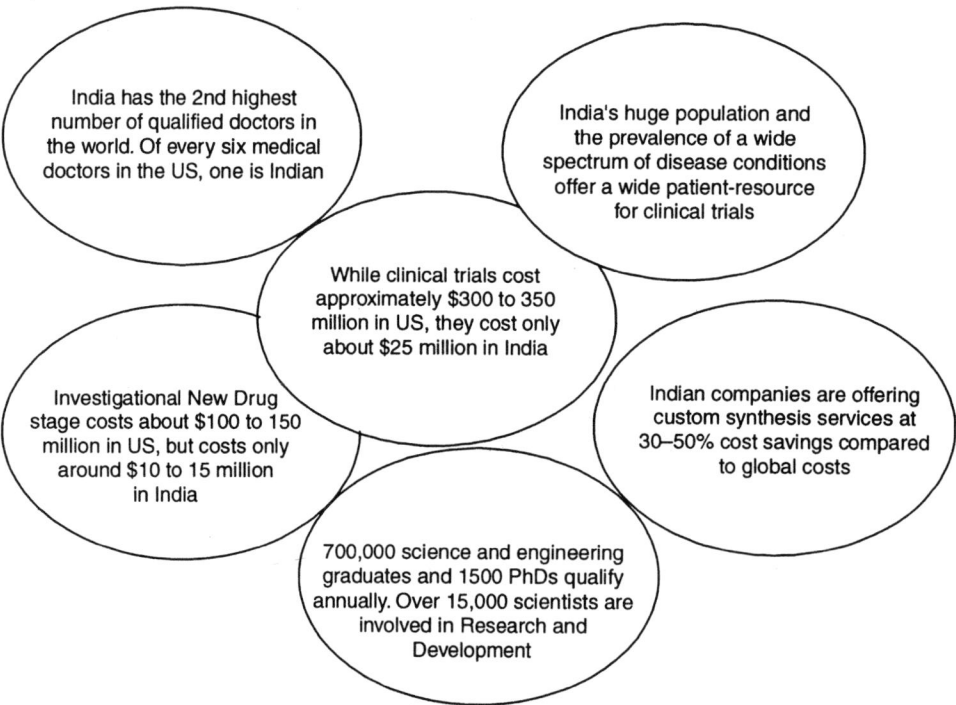

Fig. 1.9. Attractive features of India

Advantages of Outsourcing to India

- Large number of English-speaking graduates and high percentage of computer literacy
- High patient-doctor population (more patients per doctor)
- Known to have the best brains in information technology
- High calibre, dedicated scientists and clinical research professionals
- Increased enthusiasm to participate in global multicentre clinical trials and cutting-edge technology
- Government supportive of pharmaceutical and biotechnology companies
- Proposed changes to Schedule Y of Drug & Cosmetics Act, 1940 and Rules, 1945 by DCGI
- Hospitals attached to medical institutions: 164 plus other major corporate hospitals and specialized institutions

Table 1.3: India has clinical research resources on par or better vis–a–vis the world

	India vs Western countries	*India vs. China*
+	Patient enrollment Diversity Genetic uniqueness Costs	Diversity Genetic uniqueness English competency Medical infrastructure Familiarity with western medicine
=	• English competency • Medical infrastructure • Western medicine familiarity • Companies with international standards	• Costs • Patient enrollment
−	• IPR reputation • Industry standards • Less established infrastructure	• Foreign partnerships • Resources • Patent regime

Source: Presentation by Dr RS Nadig, VP. Clinigene, at the confederation of Indian Industries on 7th Feb. 2003 at N. Delhi

BIO–IT INITIATIVES

IT/ITES companies like Accenture, Wipro, Intel, Satyam, Cognizant, IBM, Oracle and TCS have ventured into offering bio-IT initiatives in India. While some of them have actively started the clinical data management initiatives, others are planning to venture in IT solutions, installation and implementation, training and familiarisation supports. For example, Pfizer, India has signed a contract with Cognizant Technologies, India seeking data capture, data management, statistics services for its phase I, II, III global trials. Similarly, Accenture is working exclusively for Wyeth in clinical trial data management. IBM Life Science solutions aims to provide the IT infrastructure that researchers in biotechnology, pharmaceutical research, genomics, proteomics, and healthcare need to turn data into scientific discovery.

Wipro's Healthcare Life Science division claims to offer pharma companies IT solutions that will reduce drug discovery and approval time. Sakti Group, a New York and Bangalore-based company is also doing data management and statistics work. Besides this, every small and big software company is developing a package/software for clinical trial management, project management, documentation management, approaching small CROs, pharma companies, etc.

JOB TRENDS IN THE CLINICAL TRIALS INDUSTRY

The Indian market is going to be flooded with plenty of job opportunities in this field. Doctors, Pharmacists, Graduates and students with science/medicine background can gain entry in this field. In a survey sponsored by Consign Med, 33.7% of the respondents replied that they work in the Pharmaceutical, Biopharmaceutical, and Biologics industry, 30.8% are involved in clinical study and/or with investigative sites, including academia and medical research faculties and 18% are involved with Contract Research Organizations. Both pharmaceutical and biotech employment are predicted to increase by the year 2012. The McKinsey report says that more than 50,000 professionals would be required to cater the needs of the industry in the near future.

EDUCATIONAL TRAINING

With increase in the popularity of clinical research, more training courses need to be offered by the Universities to meet the huge demand of highly qualified professionals so as to cater the needs of the industry. Few academic institutes in India like ICRI (with 3 centres in India), Academy of Clinical excellence (Mumbai), University of Pune, are offering certificate and diploma courses in clinical research. Recently Lotus labs, Bangalore has also started offering courses in clinical research. The bioequivalence study centre, Jadavpur University also has plans of starting courses in clinical research in the near future.

FUTURE ACTION PLAN

Since the promise for the future is big, we need to mould ourselves and sharpen our skills and expertise to make best use of the opportunities lying ahead of us.

- Build infrastructure to meet the global standards.
- Create a strong working environment compliant with the ICH, GCP, GLP Guidelines.
- Generate quality and reliable data to be approved by regulatory bodies.
- Train ourselves to attain global recognition through accreditations and certifications.
- Attain and maintain the status as the destination for clinical trials.

CONCLUSION

With India emerging as IT superpower and clinical trial hub, outsourcing to India for clinical data management is more obvious than predicted. The Indian industry, which earlier relied on its cost effectiveness to attract customers, is now moving towards an entirely different direction. Quality and fast response are the new buzzword to dominate the business processes which ensure accurate, reliable services to the customers. The need of the hour is more specialized training and education in the field of clinical research to grab the bigger opportunities. Also implementation of more stringent guidelines for conducting research on humans and strict improved functioning of Ethics committee would boost the clinical trials market in India to greater heights.

ACKNOWLEDGEMENT

We sincerely thank Medical Council of India (MCI), New Delhi for funding the seminar organized by us on Clinical Research — Practice & Prospects. This seminar was the basis for upgrading our prior knowledge on clinical trials which ultimately encouraged us to write this article.

REFERENCES

1. Susanna J Dodgson. The evolution of clinical trials. The write stuff, vol. 15, No. 1, 2006.
2. www.epresspharmaonline.com
3. www.actamagazine.com
4. www.contractpharma.com
5. www.acrohealth.org
6. www.researchandmarkets.com

Chapter 2

Ethics and Clinical Trial Management

Sangita Agarwal
T.K. Pal
T.K. Chattaraj

BACKGROUND

In traditional medical practice, the doctor prescribes a treatment based on his past experience and of others, which in his judgement is the best prognosis. Since there are few conditions for which treatment is 100% effective, there is much scope for potential improvements in therapy. Such improvements are derived via a clinical trial.

What is Clinical Trial?

Clinical Trials or **Clinical Research** is a structured process by which new pharmaceutical medicines, medical devices and biologically active agents are evaluated for safety, efficacy and utility to ascertain whether they actually help treat a disease or not. This information is required by both manufacturers, to ensure they have a viable product, and most importantly by national and international regulatory authorities to enable them to determine if a new medicine or a healthcare product is safe for general public. In reality, without clinical trials, there would be no new medicines or drugs coming in the market.

Treatments for patients affected by end-stage diseases have been developed, thanks to highly advanced diagnostic tests and new treatments. Clinicians often ask patients to participate in a clinical trial, or patients may receive information on clinical trials in progress at specialized centres. The choice to participate in a clinical trial represents an important and personal decision. Patients and their families should review all the information to make an informed decision. It is often useful to consult your family doctor with your family and friends when deciding whether or not to participate in a trial. Having identified the available open trials, the next step is to contact the research staff for information on specific trials.[1–2]

Clinical Trials —Indian Scenario

The clinical research environment has become extremely competitive and commercialized. Every year about 80,000 clinical trials conducted in the world are estimated to cost about $ 12 million. It is increasingly difficult and expensive to find enough people for Phase III clinical trials that require hundreds of thousands of participants. Dozens of Clinical Research Organizations (CROs) have suddenly proliferated in India and hundreds of hospitals, public and private, are busy carrying out industry driven clinical trials. US drug companies are moving their trials overseas, because India has no dearth of willing doctor researchers (our 162 medical colleges produce 17,000 doctors every year), who can enroll enough meek and mute patients into clinical trials to satisfy the needs of the drug and device industry. Though the Helsinki declaration explicitly states that "the interests of the subject must always prevail over the interest of science or society", the current research is being driven less by an intellectual curiosity or genuine research questions to advance science, but more by huge conflicts of interests.

In the year 2000, The Indian Council of Medical Research (ICMR) laid down comprehensive ethical guidelines within which biomedical research should function. Good Clinical Practice and Regulatory requirements for clinical trials of drugs in India laid down by CDSCO have been attached as Appendix. The council, however, lacks statutory power to ensure that they are being implemented. There are several instances where ethical norms in research in India have been clearly flouted. For example, 400 unsuspecting young women were used as guinea pigs by self styled researchers to evaluate if an anti-cancer drug, Letrozole, can also be used to induce ovulation. In the year 1994, investigators had told 10 patients (most sex workers) infected with HIV in Mumbai that they were being administered a miracle vaccine. Such unethical and illegal trials are conducted without any fear because regulatory authorities, either by design or default, fail to take action. The code of federal regulations requires that clinical trials must be "well-designed, well-conducted, performed by qualified investigators, and conducted in accordance with ethical principles acceptable to the world community".

GUIDELINES FOR ETHICAL CONDUCT OF CLINICAL TRIAL

Several agencies regulating the conduct on biomedical research have drafted useful guidelines to ensure ethical conduct of clinical trials. According to these guidelines, researchers are expected to know The Elements of Informed Consent (Table 2.1), Patient's Bill of Rights (Table 2.2) and Elements of a Consent Form (Table 2.3).

Table 2.1: Elements of informed consent

- A statement explaining the purpose of the research, the procedures to be followed, the duration of participation and any investigational treatment or procedures.
- A description of foreseeable risks or discomforts to the subjects.
- A description of benefits that the participant can reasonably expect.
- A disclosure of appropriate alternative procedures or courses of treatment that might be advantageous to the participants.
- A statement describing how confidentiality of records will be maintained.
- An explanation of compensation and whether medical treatments are available if injury occurs.
- A list of contacts to answer study related questions and to help with research-related injuries.
- A statement that participation is voluntary and that there is no penalty or loss of benefits for refusing to participate.

Additional Elements on Informed Consent Forms when Appropriate

- A statement of unforeseeable risks to the volunteer, embryo or fetus, if the volunteer is or may become pregnant.

- A list of anticipated circumstances under which the investigator may terminate a volunteer's participation.
- A description of additional costs to the volunteer.
- An explanation of consequences and procedures if a volunteer decides to withdraw.
- A statement about informing volunteers of significant new findings that might affect their willingness to participate.
- A description of the number of volunteers participating in the study.

(*Source:* Code of Federal Regulations. Title 21, Section 50.25. Partners Human Research Committee: Informed Consent of Human Subjects; February 2004)

Table 2.2: The clinical trial volunteer's bill of rights

Any volunteer who gives his or her consent to participate in a clinical trial or who is asked to give his or her consent on behalf of another has the following rights: • To be told the purpose of the clinical trial. • To be told about all the risks, side effects or discomforts that might be reasonably expected. • To be told of any benefits that can be reasonably expected. • To be told what will happen in the study and whether any procedures, drugs or devices are different than those that are used as standard medical treatment. • To be told about options available and how they may be better or worse than being in a clinical trial. • To be allowed to ask any questions about the trial before giving consent and at any time during the course of the study. • To be allowed ample time, without pressure, to decide whether to consent or not to consent to participate. • To refuse to participate, for any reason, before and after the trial has started. • To receive a signed and dated copy of the informed consent form. • To be told of any medical treatments available if complications occur during the trial.

Table 2.3: Elements of a consent form

• Title of the study	• Sponsor
• Investigator	• Study place
• Nature and purpose of the study	• Duration of the study
• Description of the study	• Risks, inconveniences and discomforts
• Safeguards	• Benefits
• Alternatives	• Costs
• Confidentiality	• Conflicts of interests
• Research related injury	• Compensation
• Withdrawal from the study	• Contact information

Thus, a clinical trial is the application of the scientific method to human health. Since such trials require the use of human test subjects and can severely impact the well-being of the subjects, as well as treatments of other people and large amounts of capital for those performing the trial, the proper **management of clinical trials** is crucial.

INTRODUCTION TO CLINICAL TRIAL MANAGEMENT

The Clinical Development of a drug is a complex and costly process which must be conducted under numerous bonds and regulations. Monitoring clinical studies, in particular, data management, is quite demanding, both in terms of the time required and the human resources dedicated to this process. Pharmaceutical companies have been trying to improve the overall quality, timeliness, and efficiency of their clinical development process. Information technology offers them an opportunity to do so. In fact, the pervasive presence of innovation due to information technology is changing the way we work, frequently faster than we would like. Pharmaceutical companies can spend 12 to 15 years and up to $900 million to bring a drug to market. About 45 percent of this cost is accrued during the clinical trial phase. Additionally, studies indicate that 75 percent of all trials conducted in the United States are behind schedule by one to six months.[3-4]

CHALLENGES IN CARRYING CLINICAL TRIALS

Improving time-to-market for new drugs is critical for pharmaceutical companies, managing the clinical trial process is one of the most significant areas of opportunity for improvement. Today, pharmaceutical companies struggle with the following challenges:

- **Lengthy and complex trial design and planning process.** Clinical trials can often involve thousands of patients and hundreds of support staff.
- **Inefficiencies and delays capturing patient data.** Consistent, streamlined capture of patient data is critical for success.
- **Inability to connect to a wide variety of systems.** Clinical trials often involve interaction with numerous trial sites using disparate systems and processes.
- **Difficulty remaining compliant with FDA guidelines.** Stringent FDA regulations are placing more pressure on how clinical trials are managed.
- **Lack of archive materials to build best practices.** Each clinical trial often is started from scratch, not utilizing historical best practices and feedback.

Overall, pharmaceutical companies will benefit from streamlining the clinical trial management process through a clinical trial management solution.

Clinical Trial Recruitment

Over the last ten years, getting patients and doctors into clinical trials has become the most delay-ridden aspect of the drug discovery and development process. When implemented effectively, clinical trial recruitment (CTR) initiatives can be highly successful. Time lines can be drammatically reduced and recruitment targets can be met ahead of schedule and every single day saved in the progression to marketing authorization, can equate to millions of pounds made in patent-protected sales revenue.

However, great care is needed in the development of a CTR program. Considerable ethical scrutiny is applied to all patient recruitment materials and initiatives. For example, in 2002 the European Commission issued guidelines for consultation which require patient advertising and details of recruitment initiatives to be submitted to appropriate ethics committees. Unfortunately, there is no simple code of practice established and no unified regulatory body and no recourse to appeal. Enhancing CTR is obviously an area in which great caution is required. Some investigating doctors, for example, question the need for extra activities as, they claim, there are sufficient number of suitable patients among those already attending their clinics. However, practical experience has shown that this is an over-estimation of the number of patients physicians will be able to recruit and it is estimated that only about 10% of a physician's patients will actually wish to enroll in a clinical trial.

Perhaps more importantly, there are also objections raised from within the industry. These usually centre on a highly cautious approach to the ethics and legitimacy of patient-facing initiatives. Some nervousness is understandable given the strict controls that govern DTC marketing but for clinical research there is a critical need for increased patient understanding and education. The signs are that the caution of the industry is slowly giving way to a new openness and confidence. A review of recent press coverage also highlights a deep skepticism of industry involvement in clinical research. If not approached ethically, a firm's CTR campaign can leave them wide open to aggressive media criticism and adverse advocacy relationships. The key point to remember is that the objective of this entire work is ultimately to improve care for the patient. A strenuous effort to maintain this focus throughout clinical development will ultimately allow pharma companies to reap considerable rewards.

Over the past several years these problems have been addressed in the US, where clinical research receives more and more active support of government bodies, advocacy groups, charities and patient groups. This provides a collaborative environment and ensures that there is always an independent counterpoint when the integrity of industry-sponsored studies is attacked.[5]

Study Designs and Methods

A common pitfall is insufficiently rigorous evaluation of study designs and methods. A "straw poll" during a clinical project management training course revealed that virtually all clinical protocols have at least one amendment during the study. The reasons appear to cover the full range, from reliance on well-established designs without allowing newer, more creative ideas to be considered and, at the other extreme, not testing new methods for the current application. For example, in a recent angina study, treadmill exercise testing was used as the primary efficacy criterion. This is, of course, extremely well-validated methodology, but, in this case, the patients were elderly, so the exercise protocol was substantially modified to reduce the physical demand. The problem was that with such a mild exercise protocol, less than half the patients recruited showed sufficient electrocardiogram (ECG) changes to qualify for randomization. A quick pilot study would have alerted the sponsors before committing to major cost.

The Role of Senior Management

A recurring theme in clinical research is the role of senior management. By this we mean not the head of clinical research, not the head of R&D, but corporate management. The costs and risks of failure in the clinical phases are so large that they should be occupying much of top management's attention. Yet, in many companies, requirements, objectives, budgets, and deadlines, are imposed without any negotiation. On top of this, major changes are commonly dictated by management, usually by changing priorities. How can the clinical project manager fulfil top management's aspirations, within an increasingly constrained environment?

Risk Management

All research and development normally involves some risk. Some of the risks are typically encountered in the main stages of a typical clinical trial. The values for risk level and lateness are those usually applied in our company when planning studies. They are useful rules of thumb. Whatever rules are used, they will almost certainly be better than no risk assessment at all.

The assessment of risks and benefits requires a careful description of relevant data, including, in some cases alternative ways of obtaining the benefits sought in the research. Thus, the assessment presents both an opportunity and a responsibility to gather systematic and comprehensive information about proposed research. Patients who volunteer for medical research can face risks over and above those normally encountered in their everyday lives. The degree of such risks can often be known only after the research has been completed. Professional pressure can lead researchers to underestimate inconvenience and hazard, misleading volunteers in the process. Volunteers must have accurate and detailed information about potential risks in order to protect themselves. To deny volunteers such information is a clear breach of their moral rights. Some researchers argue that informed consent may not be necessary for studies where invasiveness and risks are negligible.

They also believe that participants, distressed by detailed information about risks involved in a trial may panic, which may compromise their subsequent doctor-patient relationship, and may keep patients form entering trials in sufficient numbers to make such trials possible. Too much emphasis on the rights of individuals, researchers feel, may put hurdles in the growth of science. Patients receiving medical care, according to them, have a duty to promote further research for future generations. If the volunteers discover that information has been withheld, their distress and sense of betrayal may be far greater than that engendered by learning the truth. Even those patients who are terminally ill want accurate information and are not necessarily upset by it. Participants in medical research are unlikely to get distressed by knowing unpleasant facts and have a right to know all details before they say yes.

ICMR guidelines clearly stipulate that volunteers must be provided all information on physical and psychological risks as well as moral implications of the research. They also state that research should include an in-built mechanism for compensation to cover "all foreseeable and unforeseeable risks" a fact rarely mentioned in most consent forms. Research involving human subjects and biological sciences poses complex ethical issues. It requires careful thought and consideration on the part of both researcher and research participants.

Risk Distribution in Clinical Phases

Delivering the results on time, to the required standard, may have a lower risk in phase I than in later phases, mainly because subjects are healthy and not potentially complicated patients, and thus, recruitment can be predicted with some confidence. However, first administration to humans is something of a leap into the unknown, and safety problems are always to be considered. What is possibly less obvious is the risk of any early-phase design errors to later phases and to the whole drug project. Once phase III is imminent, perhaps there is a degree of confidence emerging, as much more is known about the drug. The requirement for phase III, therefore, may be seen as accumulating data to enable a product license application. In fact, the great expansion of activity dictated by phase III studies introduces even more complexity and a new set of risks. The application of the drug to a more realistic clinical setting means that we will not necessarily by studying "clean" patients. Patients will often have other diseases on top of that under study and will only be under observation for a small proportion of the time. Attention to clinical protocol design, thus, is at least as critical as in phases I-II.

Key Tasks

The most common reason for late tasks and projects is that they are started late. Before patients can be screened for entry, a well-established set of start-up tasks must be completed, and of these, some are relatively easy to plan, and others are less predictable. Those relying on internal agreements, e.g. drug supplies, protocol sign-off, can be expedited by instilling the right culture of negotiation between departments and individuals.

External Elements —Regulatory and Ethics Approvals

Regulatory approval is reasonably easy to plan, because, in most countries, there are clear limits to the time and effort required to meet regulatory requirements. Much more difficult is the matter of approval of ethical standards. Across the EU, as well as in Australia, Canada, and USA, ethics committees' practices may vary enormously so that, when planning a multinational study, good local knowledge is crucial. Even inside the borders of the same country or state there is often inconsistency, especially since the demise of single central approval for multi-center studies. Theoretically, local research ethics committees (IRBs) are expected to follow Department of Health guidelines, but, if they choose not to do so, there is apparently no redress, so one may be presented with unexpected delays in particular centers because of widely varying IRBs' practices. There is a move toward rationalization in the form of a two-level approval process. A central committee will review the study and, if approved, pass it on to local committees for ratification.

Within the US, the Institutional Review Board (IRB) has clearly defined responsibilities and reporting lines. In Australia, central approval is still possible, and the ethics committee sees itself more as a partner in research than as regulator; the very rapid start-up of studies is possible. The message here is that, if compelling reasons to conduct one's studies in any particular country are not available, be creative with your planning, and consider the big advantages you might gain in another part of the world. If you are forced to work around the conditions outlined above, obtain the best and most recent information you can from the ECs/IRBs and from their users, and build this realistically into your plans. The results may not be to your idealization, but you will have a better chance of keeping to them.

WHAT IS A CLINICAL TRIAL MANAGEMENT SYSTEM?

A **Clinical Trial Management System**, also known as CTMS, is a customizeable software system used by the biotechnology and pharmaceutical industries to manage the large amounts of data involved with the operation of a clinical trial. It maintains and manages the planning, preparation, performance, and reporting of clinical trials, with emphasis on keeping up-to-date contact information for participants and tracking deadlines and milestones such as those for regulatory approval or the issue of progress reports. Often, a clinical trial management system provides data to a business intelligence system, which acts as a digital dashboard for trial managers.[6–7]

In the early phases of clinical trials, when the number of patients and tests are small, most managers use an in-house or home-grown program to handle their data. As the amount of data grows, though, organizations increasingly look to replace their systems with more stable, feature-rich software provided by specialized vendors. Each manager has different requirements that a system must satisfy. Some popular requirements include budgeting, patient management, compliance with government regulations, and compatibility with other data management systems.

Each sponsor has different requirements that their CTMS must satisfy; it would be impossible to create a complete list of CTMS requirements. Despite differences, several requirements are pervasive, including project management, budgeting and financials, patient management, investigator management, EC/IRB approvals, compliance with FDA regulations, and compatibility with other systems such as data management systems, electronic data capture, and adverse event reporting systems.

Objectives of the CTMS

The goal of a clinical trial management solution is to facilitate the planning, execution, and tracking of relevant clinical trial activities (Fig. 2.1). A clinical trial management solution provides the following benefits:

Improved Process Planning

- Design and prototype trials faster and easier
- Model visit schedules, data schema, edit checks, and form design using a drag-and-drop interface
- Build powerful form libraries and collaboration processes to facilitate even faster design cycle

Standardized Data Collection Processes

- Increase the speed and accuracy of data entry and exchange through Web-based data collection
- Generate more consistent reports through an FDA-compliant library of templates
- Provide single sign-on access to multiple clinical processes including electronic data capture (EDC), data management, and adverse events reporting

More Effective Data Management and Analysis

- Provide one centralized place to track progress by study, site, and staff member
- Exchange protocol synopsis, confidentiality agreements, and other critical documents electronically and securely
- Integrate with different site systems for faster data exchange, query resolution, and data reconciliation
- Provide the pharmaceutical sponsor of the trial with greater visibility of clinical data

Improved Trial Administration

- Streamline administrative processes through one central location for tasks, issues, and schedules

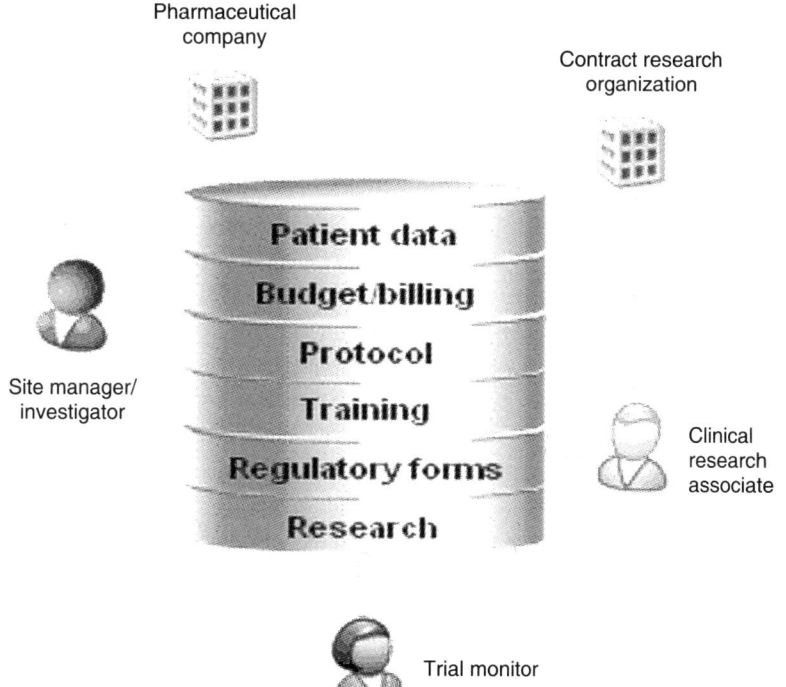

Fig. 2.1. Clinical trial management solution gathers and centralizes data

- Integrate with budgeting and finance applications
- Get team members up and running faster with both real-time and archived online training modules
- Provide sites with online access to sponsor and CRO information, archived documents, and frequently asked questions (FAQs)

The following graphic shows how a clinical trial management solution (CTMs) gathers and centralizes data for easier access, greater visibility, and more efficient processing.

Overall Advantages of using a CTMS

A solution built with the clinical trial management solution enables pharmaceutical companies to more effectively and efficiently implement and realize:

- Faster trial design and planning processes.
- More efficient collection and management of both patient and trial administration data.
- Improved FDA compliance.
- Secure, centralized access to sites, trials, and programs.
- Reduced administrative costs.

REFERENCES

1. Chow S-C and Liu JP (2004). Design and Analysis of Clinical Trials : Concepts and Methodologies, ISBN 0-471-24985-8.
2. Pocock SJ (2004), Clinical Trials: A Practical Approach, John Wiley & Sons, ISBN 0-471-90155-5
3. Choi B, Drozdetski S, Hackett M, Lu C, Rottenberg C, Yu L, Hunscher D, Clauw D., Usability comparison of three clinical trial management systems, AMIA Annu Symp Proc. 2005;:921.
4. Payne PR, Greaves AW, Kipps TJ., CRC Clinical Trials Management System (CTMS): an integrated information management solution for collaborative clinical research, AMIA Annu Symp Proc. 2003;:967.
5. Stuart Summerhayes, CDM Regulations Procedures Manual, Blackwell Publishing, ISBN 1-4051-0740-5
6. Tai BC, Seldrup J., A review of software for data management, design and analysis of clinical trials, Ann Acad Med Singapore. 2000 Sep;29(5):576-81.
7. Greenes RA, Pappalardo AN, Marble CW, Barnett GO., Design and implementation of a clinical data management system, Comput Biomed Res. 1969 Oct;2(5):469-85.

STATEMENT OF SPECIFIC PRINCIPLES FOR CLINICAL EVALUATION OF DRUGS/VACCINES/DEVICES/DIAGNOSTICS/HERBAL REMEDIES, ETC.

Human studies designed to evaluate the safety, effectiveness, or usefulness of an intervention include research on therapeutics, diagnostic procedures and preventive measures including vaccines. The type of experimental procedures that a patient is submitted to has become more complex and varied as the complexities of medical research have increased. It is clearly accepted that it is essential to carry out research on human subjects to discover better medical and therapeutic modalities for the benefit of mankind. It is equally clear that such research on normal subjects and patients is associated with some degree of risk to the individual concerned. These guidelines have been framed to carry out the evaluation of drugs, vaccines, devices and other diagnostic materials on human subjects including herbal remedies, in accordance with the basic ethical principles. These guidelines are important for the protection of research subjects against any avoidable risk and to guide the researchers in the preparation of research proposals/protocols.

For the clinical evaluation of proposed research intervention, the framework of guidelines is provided for the following areas:

1. Drug trials
2. Vaccine trials
3. Surgical procedures/medical devices
4. Diagnostic agents, with special reference to use of radioactive materials and X-rays
5. Trials with herbal remedies

GENERAL PRINCIPLES

All the research involving human subjects should be conducted in accordance with the four basic ethical principles, namely Autonomy or respect for person / subject, Beneficence, Non-maleficence and Justice. The guidelines laid down are directed at application of these basic principles to research involving human subjects. An investigator is the person responsible for the research trial and for protection of the rights, health and welfare of the subjects recruited for the study. He/she should have qualification and competence in clinical trial research methods for proper conduct of the trial and should be aware of and comply with all requirements of the study protocol as enumerated under the General Principles and General Issues.

SPECIFIC PRINCIPLES

1. Drug Trials

Clinical trial of drugs is a randomised single or double blind controlled study in human subjects, designed to evaluate prospectively the safety and effectiveness of new drugs/new formulations. The new drug as defined under the Drugs and Cosmetic Rules 1945 (OCR), and subsequent amendments include:

(*a*) a new chemical entity (NCE);
(*b*) a drug which has been approved for a certain indication, by a certain route, in a certain dosage

regimen, but which is now proposed to be used for another indication, by another route, or in another dosage regimen;

(*c*) a combination of two or more drugs which, although approved individually, are proposed to be combined for the first time in a fixed dose combination (FDC).

The proposed trial should be carried out, only after approval of the Drugs Controller General of India (DCGI), as is necessary under The Schedule Y of Drugs and Cosmetics Act, 1940. The investigator should also get the approval of Ethical Committee of the Institution before submitting the proposal to DCGI. All the guiding principles should be followed irrespective of whether the drug has been developed in this country or abroad or whether clinical trials have been carried out outside India or not.[1-2]

PHASES OF CLINICAL TRIALS[1-2]

The first three of the following four phases of clinical trials of drug require ethical clearance:—

Phase I — The objective of phase I of clinical trial is to determine the safety of the maximum tolerated dose in healthy adults of both sexes. Healthy female volunteers could be included, provided they have completed their family or do not intend to have a child in the future. At least two subjects should be administered each dose to establish the safe dose range, pharmacokinetic, pharmacodynamic effects, and adverse reactions, if any, with their intensity and nature. Investigator trained in clinical pharmacology should preferably carry out these studies. The duration of time lapsing between two trials in the same volunteer should be a minimum of 3 months. The volunteers should preferably be covered under some insurance scheme.

Phase II — These are controlled studies conducted in a limited number of patients of both sexes to determine therapeutic uses, effective dose range and further evaluation of safety and pharmacokinetics when necessary. Normally 20–25 patients should be studied for assessment of each dosage. These studies are usually limited to 3–4 centres.

Phase III — The purpose of these trials is to obtain adequate data about the efficacy and safety of drugs in a larger number of patients of both sexes in multiple centres usually in comparison with a standard drug and/or a placebo if a standard drug does not exist for the disease under study. On successful completion of phase in trials permission is granted for marketing of the drug.

Phase IV — After approval of the drug for marketing, phase IV study or post marketing surveillance is undertaken to obtain additional information about the drug's risks, benefits and optimal use. Although this is outside the purview of the ethical committee, it is an important aspect of drug trial on the long-term effects of the drugs and the adverse reactions induced by drugs, if any, should be brought to the notice of the Ethics Committee.

Throughout the drug trials, the distinction between therapy and research should be maintained. A physician/investigator who participates in research by administering the new drug to consenting patients should ensure that the patients understand and remember that the drug is experimental and that its benefits for the condition under study are yet unproven. Use of a placebo in drug trials and sham surgery has come under severe scrutiny at the present age and requires careful consideration before approval. Denial of the available treatment to control (placebo) group of patients is unethical.

- Trials of drugs without the approval of the appropriate authority should be dealt according to the law of the land and the guidelines formulated by the country's regulatory agencies.

- After the clinical trial is over, if need be, it should be made mandatory that the sponsoring agency should provide the drug to the patient till it is marketed in the country.
- The criteria for termination of a trial must be defined a priori in the proposal of the trial and plan of interim analysis must be clearly presented. This is important when on interim analysis the test drug is found to be clearly more effective or less effective than the standard drug. The trial can be discontinued thereafter and better drug should be given to patient receiving less effective drug.
- Issues of partner notification and discordant couples should be taken care of before initiating any HIV/AIDS related trial.

Good Clinical Practices (GCP) provide operative guidelines for ethical and scientific standards for the designing of a trial protocol including conduct, recording and reporting procedures and should be strictly adhered to while carrying out a trial. Till such time that the Standard Operating Procedures (SOP) for Indian GCP are formulated, the international guidelines issued by World Health Organization (WHO) and International Committee on Harmonization (ICH) should be followed.

SPECIAL CONCERNS

1. Multicentric Trials

A multicentric trial is conducted simultaneously by several investigators at different centres following the same protocol and pro formae. Ideally, these trials should be initiated at the same time at all the centres.

- All the investigators should give a written acceptance of the protocol to be followed for the trial duly approved by the ethics committee of the host institutes.
- Meetings should be organised at the initial and intermediary stages of the trial to ensure uniform procedures at all centres.
- Training should be imparted to research staff at the participating centres to familiarize them with the uniform procedures.
- Standardisation of methods for recruitment and evaluation/monitoring of laboratory procedures and conduct of trial should be carried out.
- There should be monitoring of adherence to protocol including measures to terminate the participation of some centres, if necessary.
- Specific role of coordinators and monitors should be defined.
- Centralised data management and analysis should be planned.
- Drafting of a common final report and publication procedure should be decided at the outset
- No individual centre should publish any data till appropriate authorities accept the combined report.
- The code of the administered drug could be broken in the event of a severe adverse reaction occurring during the conduct of a double blind trial necessitating such a step.

MONITORING AND REPORTING ADVERSE REACTIONS OR EVENTS

Any serious adverse events occurring during the course of the trial should be immediately brought to the attention of ethics committee, sponsors and Drug Controller General of India. At the end of the trial, all adverse events, whether related to trial or not, are to be listed, evaluated and discussed in detail in the final report.

DATA REQUIRED TO BE SUBMITTED WITH APPLICATION FOR PERMISSION TO MARKET A NEW DRUG

1. Introduction
A brief description of the drug and the therapeutic class to which it belongs.

2. Chemical and Pharmaceutical Information
1. Chemical name; code name or number, if any; non-proprietary or generic name, if any; physio-chemical proportion
2. Dosage form and its composition
3. Specifications of active and inactive ingredients
4. Tests for identification of the active ingredient and method of its assay
5. Outline of the method of manufacture of the active ingredient
6. Stability data.

3. Animal Pharmacology
1. Summary
2. Specific pharmacological actions
3. General pharmacological actions
4. Pharmacokinetics, absorptions, distribution, metabolism, excretion.

4. Animal Toxicology
1. Summary
2. Acute toxicity
3. Long-term toxicity
4. Reproduction studies
5. Local toxicity
6. Mutagenicity and carcinogenicity.

5. Human/Clinical Pharmacology (Phase I)
1. Summary
2. Specific pharmacological actions
3. General pharmacological actions
4. Pharmacokinetics, absorptions, distribution, metabolism, excretion.

6. Exploratory Clinical Trials (Phase II)
1. Summary
2. Investigator wise reports.

7. Confirmatory Clinical Trials (Phase III)
1. Summary
2. Investigator wise reports.

8. Special Studies

1. Summary
2. Bioavailability and dissolution studies
3. Investigator wise reports.

9. Regulatory Status in Other Countries

1. Countries where
   (*a*) Marketed
   (*b*) Approved
   (*c*) Under trial, with phase
   (*d*) Withdrawn, if any, with reasons

2. Restrictions on use, if any, in countries where marketed/approved
3. Free sale certificate from country of origin.

10. Marketing Information

1. Proposed product monograph
2. Drafts of labels and cartons
3. Sample of pure drug substance, with testing protocol.

Notes I: All items may not be applicable to all drugs, for explanation, see text of Schedule Y.

II: For requirements of data to be submitted with application for clinical trials see text of Schedule Y, Section I and also Appendices II and III to Sch. Y.

Appendix X

CONTENTS OF THE PROPOSED PROTOCOL FOR CONDUCTING CLINICAL TRIALS

1. TITLE PAGE

(*a*) Full title of the clinical study
(*b*) Protocol/and protocol version number with date
(*c*) The IND name/number of the investigational drug·
(*d*) Complete name and address of the sponsor and contract research organization, if any
(*e*) List of the investigators who are conducting the study, their respective institutional affiliations and site locations
(*f*) Name(s) of clinical laboratories and other departments and/or faculties participating in the study.

2. TABLE OF CONTENTS

A complete Table of Contents including a list of all Appendices.

1. Background and Introduction

(*a*) Preclinical experience
(*b*) Clinical experience

Previous clinical work with the new drug should be reviewed here and a description of how the current protocol extends existing data should be provided. If this is an entirely new indication, how this drug was considered for this should be discussed. Relevant information regarding pharmacological, toxicological and other biological properties of the drug/biological/medical device, and previous efficacy and safety experience should be described.

2. Study Rationale

This section should describe a brief summary of the background information relevant to the study design and protocol methodology. The reasons for performing this study in the particular population included by the protocol should be provided.

3. Study Objective(s) (Primary as well as Secondary) and Their Logical Relation to the Study Design

3. STUDY DESIGN

   (*a*) Overview of the Study Design: Including a description of the type of study (i.e. double blind, multicentre, placebo controlled, etc.) a detail of the specific treatment groups and number of study subjects in each group and investigative site, subject number assignment, and the type, sequence and duration of study periods.
   (*b*) Flow chart of the study.
   (*c*) Discussion of Study Design: This discussion details the rationale for the design chosen for this study.

   1. Study population: The number of subjects required to be enrolled in the study at the investigative site and by all sites along with a brief description of the nature of the subject population required is also mentioned.
   2. Subject eligibility

      (*a*) Inclusion criteria
      (*b*) Exclusion criteria

   3. Study Assessments: Plan, procedures and methods to be described in detail.
   4. Study Conduct stating the types of study activities that would be included in this section would be: medical history, type of physical examination, blood or urine testing, electrocardiogram (ECG), diagnostic testing such as pulmonary function tests, symptom measurement, dispensation and retrieval of medication, subject cohort assignment, adverse event review, etc.
   Each visit should be described separately as Visit 1, Visit 2, etc.
   Discontinued Subjects: Describes the circumstances for Subject withdrawal, dropouts, or other reasons for discontinuation of subjects, state how dropouts would be managed and if they would be replaced.
   Describe the method of handling of protocol waivers, if any. The person(s) who approves all such waivers should be identified and the criteria used for specific waivers should be provided. Describes how protocol violations will be treated, including conditions where the study will be terminated for non-compliance with the protocol.
   5. Study Treatment

      (*a*) Dosing schedule (dose, frequency, and duration of the experimental treatment). Describes the administration of placebos and/or dummy medications if they are part of the treatment plan. If applicable, concomitant drug(s), their doses, frequency, and duration of concomitant treatment should be stated.

(*b*) Study drug supplies and administration: A statement about who is going to provide the study medication and that the investigational drug formulation has been manufactured following all regulations details of the product stability, storage requirements and dispensing requirements should be provided.

(*c*) Dose modification for study drug toxicity: Rules for changing the dose or stopping the study drug should be provided.

(*d*) Possible drug interactions

(*e*) Concomitant therapy: The drugs that are permitted during the study and the conditions under which they may be used are detailed here. Describes the drugs that a subject is not allowed to use during parts of or the entire study. If any washout periods for prohibited medications are needed prior to enrollment, these should be described here.

(*f*) Blinding procedures: A detailed description of the blinding procedure if the study employs a blind on the investigator and/or the subject.

(*g*) Unblinding procedures: If the study is blinded, the circumstances in which unblinding may be done and the mechanism to be used for unblinding should be given.

6. Adverse Events (See Appendix XI): Description of expected adverse events should be given. Procedures used to evaluate an adverse event should be described.

7. Ethical Considerations: Give the summary of:

(*a*) Risk/benefit assessment

(*b*) Ethics committee review and communications

(*c*) Informed consent process

(*d*) Statement of subject confidentiality including ownership of data and coding procedures

8. Study Monitoring and Supervision: A description of study monitoring policies and procedures should be provided along with the proposed frequency of site monitoring visits, and who is expected to perform monitoring.

Case Record Form (CRF) completion requirements, including who gets which copies of the forms and any specifics required in filling out the forms CRF correction requirements, including who is authorized to make corrections on the CRF and how queries about study data are handled and how errors, if any, are to be corrected should be stated.

Investigator study files, including what needs to be stored following study completion should be described.

9. Investigational Product Management

(*a*) Give investigational product description and packaging (stating all ingredients and the formulation of the investigation of drug and any placebos used in the study)

(*b*) The precise dosing required during the study

(*c*) Method of packaging, labeling, and blinding of study substances

(*d*) Method of assigning treatments to subjects and the subject identification code numbering system

(*e*) Storage conditions for study substances

(*f*) Investigational product accountability: Describe instructions for the receipt, storage, dispensation, and return of the investigational products to ensure a complete accounting of all investigational products received, dispensed, and returned/destroyed.

(*g*) Describe policy and procedure for handling unused investigational products.

10. Data Analysis

    Provide details of the statistical approach to be followed including sample size, how the sample size was determined, including assumptions made in making this determination, efficacy endpoints (primary as well as secondary) and safety endpoints.

    Statistical analysis: Give complete details of how the results will be analyzed and reported along with the description of statistical tests to be used to analyze the primary and secondary endpoints defined above. Describe the level of significance, statistical tests to be used, and the methods used for missing data; method of evaluation of the data for treatment failures, non-compliance, and subject withdrawals; rationale and conditions for any interim analysis, if planned.

    Describe statistical considerations for Pharmacokinetic (PK) analysis, if applicable

11. Undertaking by the investigator (see Appendix VII)

12. Appendices: Provide a study synopsis, copies of the informed consent documents (patient information sheet, informed consent form, etc.); CRF and other data collection forms; a summary of relevant pre-clinical safety information and any other documents referenced in the clinical protocol.

Appendix XI

DATA ELEMENTS FOR REPORTING SERIOUS ADVERSE EVENTS OCCURRING IN A CLINICAL TRIAL

1. Patient Details

    Initials and other relevant identifier (hospital/OPD record number, etc.)*
    Gender
    Age and/or date of birth
    Weight
    Height

2. Suspected Drug(s)

    Generic name of the drug*
    Indication(s) for which suspected drug was prescribed or tested
    Dosage form and strength
    Daily dose and regimen (specify units, e.g. mg, ml, mg/kg)
    Route of administration
    Starting date and time of day
    Stopping date and time, or duration of treatment

3. Other Treatment(s)

    Provide the same information for concomitant drugs (including non-prescription/OTC drugs) and non-drug therapies, as for the suspected drug(s).

4. Details of Suspected Adverse Drug Reaction(s)

    Full description of reaction(s) including body site and severity, as well as the criterion (or criteria) for regarding the report as serious. In addition to, whenever possible, describe a specific diagnosis for the reaction.*

Start date (and time) of onset of reaction
Stop date (and time) or duration of reaction
Dechallenge and rechallenge information
Setting e.g. hospital, out-patient clinic, home, nursing home

5. Outcome
Information on recovery and any sequelae; results of specific tests and/or treatment that may have been conducted for a fatal outcome, cause of death and a comment on its possible relationship to the suspected reaction; Any post-mortem findings.
Other information: anything relevant to facilitate assessment of the case, such as medical history including allergy, drug or alcohol abuse, family history; findings from special investigations, etc.

6. Details about the Investigator*
Name
Address
Telephone number
Profession (speciality)
Date of reporting the event to Licensing Authority
Date of reporting the event to Ethics Committee overseeing the site
Signature of the Investigator
Note: Information marked * must be provided.
(F.No. X-11014/1/2003-DMS & PFA)
(RITA TEOTIA),
JOINT SECRETARY, GOVERNMENT OF INDIA

REFERENCES

1. Good Clinical Practice & Regulatory Requirements for Clinical trials in India; Central Drugs Standard Central Organisation, India 2001.
2. Schedule Y, 2005, Good Clinical Practice & Regulatory Requirements for Clinical trials in India; Central Drugs Standard Central Organisation, India.

The Prinicipal Rules were published in the Official Gazette vide notification No. F. 28-10/45-Hd), dated the 21st December, 1945 and last amended vide G.S.R. (E) dated 13-12-2004.

Chapter 3

Contract Research Industry: *An Overview*

Umakanta Sahoo

India, at the moment, is the most preferred destination for clinical research because of its heterogeneous huge patient population; English-speaking western educated investigators (physicians) and track record of sincerity in meeting regulatory and recruitment timelines, and most importantly well-accepted good quality auditable data. While the global pharmaceutical companies are increasing their clinical trial investments in India, many small and big regional pharma companies are considering India in their drug development initiatives. There is a perceptible change in the old mindset of people — from skepticism to acceptance — of the capability, skill-sets and quality of data in Indian trials.

Cost-effectiveness, competition and the increased confidence on capabilities and skill sets have propelled many global pharmaceutical players (Pfizer, Novartis, Astra Zeneca, Eli Lilly, GSK, Aventis, Novo Nordisk, etc.) to expand their own clinical research investment and infrastructure in India. Evaluating the business progression and futuristic projections of top notch services firm like Ernst & Young, McKinsey, Strategic Associates, etc, while global pharmaceutical companies and Contract Research Organisations (CRO) are opening up their branches / offices, the small biotech, pharmaceutical and Research and Development (R&D) companies are looking for preferred partners to conduct their research activities in India. The report captures the striking regulatory change, i.e. the amendment of Schedule Y (2005), which is a step towards harmonizing the Indian regulatory framework with international Good Clinical Practice (GCP) for all the stakeholders in clinical research including the sponsors, CROs, Site Management Organisations (SMOs), Institutional Ethics Committees (IECs), Investigators and the subjects participating in clinical trials in India.

The Players

Today India is moving firmly into the front ranks of the rapidly growing Asia Pacific economy and is witnessing a radical change as a business hub for clinical research.[1] Over the past decade, several players have begun to operate in several ancillary business segments of clinical research. Some of these are highlighted in the Table 3.1.

Although these players have already started operating in India, still there are a number of concerns centered on infrastructure, facilities, regulations, patents, health insurance and few of them have been addressed in this article.

Table 3.1: Clinical Research Players

Types	*Players*
Contract Research Organisation	Quintiles, Chiltern, PPD, Covance, Pharmanet, Parexel, ICON, Kendle, Pharm Olam, IGate, PRA International, Inversk, SIRO, Synchron, ClinInvent, Sterling, Clingene, ClinWorld, ClinRx, Clintec, PharmaIntel, ACT/Suven, Reliance, Apothecaries, Clinquest, Indigene, RxMD, Helix, KARD Scientific, GVK Bio
Bioequivalence and Bioanalytical Trials	Synchron, Lambda Therapeutics, Lotus Lab, Vimta Lab, Wellquest, Jubilant, LG Lifescience, Phoenix, Oxygen, Therapeutic Drug Monitoring, ClinSearch, Ace Biomed, Bio-assay, Reliance, PERD Centre, Medlar
Site Management Organisation	Neeman Medical, Odyssey Research, Accunova, Metropolis, Quintiles Patient Recruitment Organisation ICRI Synexus
Data Management and ITES Business	Quintiles, Chiltern, Synchron, Cognizant, SIRO, Accenture, DnO, ClinInvent, TCS, IBM, HCL, Infosys, Persistent Technologies, Sristek
Central Laboratories Services	Specialty Ranbaxy, Clinigene International, Metropolis Health Services, Max Healthcare, Dr Lal's Pathlab, Pathnet, Thyrocare, Lambda Therapeutics
Centralised ECG Services	Quintiles, SIRO - Spacelabs
CR Training Institutes	Academy of Clinical Excellence, Catalyst Clinical Services, Institute of Clinical Research INDIA, Kundnani College of Pharmacy, SIES College of Management, Kriger, Bio-informatics Institute, PEXA

Source: Chiltern International Private Limited

The Global Concerns

Eastern Europe was a preferred destination for clinical research in last few years because of the advantage of low cost and fast recruitment potential. Now the attention from Eastern Europe is diverted to other locations, because of rapid escalation of cost in this region arising out of fierce competition amongst the sponsors/contract research organizations and increased expectation of the clinical research professionals. Hence, European and USA pharmaceutical majors are now seriously looking at Asian and African countries to speed up their drug development process. While they are highly enthusiastic of carrying out high quality research in Asia and Africa, they still have a list of concerns besides the distance and time difference.

Over the last few years, India has proved to be most advantageous in comparison to other Asian and African countries, *because of its heterogeneous huge patient population, English-speaking western educated investigators (physicians) and track record of sincerity in meeting regulatory and recruitment timelines, and most importantly well-accepted good quality auditable data.* This chapter delves into the expectations of the global fraternity and attempts to address many common questions regarding disease prevalence pattern, regulatory framework and guidelines, health infrastructure, regulatory submissions and approval timelines, health insurance, protection of intellectual property and patent systems in India.

Disease Prevalence and Recruitment Projections

India is a vast country with 1065 million populations. There are 2–2.5 million cancer patients, over 35 million cardiac patients, 30–35 million diabetic patients and 3.8–4.5 million HIV/AIDS patients. These huge numbers are essentially estimates based on prevalence / incidence rates. Besides, there are huge numbers of patients in all other therapeutic areas. Based on the feasibility and the past experience of many global multi-centric phase II and III studies, the author informed interested parties that most studies in India have the potential to recruit 4–5 times higher and faster than any center in Europe and USA. He informed them that even some of the difficult diseases in the Oncology area, could recruit 200 patients in a less than 2 years of recruitment time from less than 10 centers. This recruitment becomes possible only through referral network and without any campaign and advertisement.

Clinical Trial Infrastructure

Besides huge recruitment potential, India has 14,000 general hospitals, of which around 150 have served as sites for clinical trials in the recent years. Most studies are done in medical colleges and hospitals. Studies are also carried out in private hospitals (like Apollo, Sterling and Manipal hospitals) and clinics. Most of these hospitals have state-of-the-art infrastructures and instruments to perform the rigorous tests and procedures in a clinical trial.

Table 3.2: Resource pool, India

Professionals	*Number*
Physicians	600,000
Nurses	737,000
Pharmacists	400,000
Medical Graduates	17,000 plus per year
Pharmacy Graduates	20,000 plus per year
Biosciences Graduates	3,000,000 plus
Biosciences Postgraduates	700,000 plus
Ph Ds in Science Stream	1500 plus

Sources: Medical Council of India, CIA World Fact Book

There are 600,000 physisians practising in these hospitals and clinics. The Medical Council of India (MCI) awards postgraduate degree per year in cardiology (75), neurology (62) and oncology (21) (Table 3.2). Hence, in super-specialty areas, currently there are around 2500 cardiologists, 2000 psychiatrists, 500 neurologists, 500 oncologists and 400 diabetologists. The majority of physicians and super specialists have increased awareness about the international clinical trials and are inclined and motivated to be part of the international studies. The standards of treatment and healthcare practices in India are lauded by global medical fraternity considering the capabilities, knowledge level and western education of these Investigators supported by their ability to speak good English and publish good research papers. Besides, there are a few central laboratories in India, which have national and international accreditation. The news of NHS in the UK considering Specialty Ranbaxy for analyzing samples of British patients, suggests that these laboratories have the credentials to be considered as central laboratory for the clinical trial.

Regulatory Framework and Guidelines

India started its voyage into global GCP trials in the last decade, when the country had no clear cut regulatory guidelines. Till then, because of pressure from the industry and proactive initiatives of the regulators, Central Ethics Committee on Human Research (CECHR) of the Indian Council of Medical Research (ICMR), New Delhi issued "Ethical Guidelines for Biomedical Research on Human Subjects" in 2000. Subsequently in 2001, a central expert committee was set up by Central Drugs Standard Control Organization (CDSCO) to develop our own Indian GCP Guidelines in line with the latest WHO, ICH, USFDA, MHRA guidelines.[2-3]

There are other proactive government policies in recent times such as revised schedule Y to allow concurrent phase trials, implementing patent Act starting January 2005, and stringent regulations to deal with spurious drug manufacturers, mandatory GMP compliance further supports the clinical development initiatives. Indian GCP guidelines and amended schedule Y 2005 (of the Drugs and Cosmetics Act) are available on CDSCO websites, www.cdsco.nic.in. The removal of phase lag in the new schedule Y is a right trend in facilitating global studies, but this is not true in case of Phase I study.

For new drug substances discovered in India, clinical trials are required to be carried out in India right from Phase I and data should be submitted to the Licensing Authority. For new drug substances discovered in countries other than India, Phase I data from other countries should be submitted along with the application. After submission of *Phase I data generated outside India to the Licensing Authority*, permission shall be granted to conduct Phase II trials and subsequently Phase III trials concurrently with other global trials for that drug. Phase III trials are required to be conducted in India before permission to market the drug in India is granted.

Regulatory and EC Approval Time

Indian regulatory framework allows concurrent submission of applications for regulatory and ethics committee (EC) approval. Clinical trial on a new drug is initiated only after the Licensing Authority (Drugs Controller General of India – DCGI) has granted the permission, and the approval obtained from the respective ethics committee(s) of the site(s). Application for permission to undertake clinical trials shall be made in Form 44 and data specified in Appendices of the Schedule Y (amended 2005) of the Drugs and Cosmetics Act, 1940 are to be submitted to the DCGI along with the application for import of new drugs. The DCGI's office takes 8 to 12 weeks for giving the regulatory approval for conduct of clinical trial in India.

Concurrently, the essential documents including translation of informed consent form and patient information sheets are submitted to the institutional EC. Most of the institutional EC meet once in a month and need the documents to be submitted 1 week prior to the meeting. The EC approval letter is issued within 1 week after the meeting. There are a few centralized EC in India and most of the Investigators prefer to have the EC approval from their institutional EC, unless the study is done in private clinic where the Investigators go to the centralized EC. The schedule Y allows the site(s) to accept the approval granted to the protocol by the ethics committee of another trial site or the approval granted by an independent ethics committee, provided that the approving ethics committee(s) is/are willing to accept their responsibilities for the study at such trial site(s) and the trial site(s) is/are willing to accept such an arrangement and that the protocol version is same at all trial sites.

Hence, regulatory permission and EC approvals are available within 8–12 weeks of submission of completed application.

Import Permission and Processes Time

The application for import of drugs is required to be made concurrently with the regulatory permission letter to DCGI. The application needs to be made in Form 12 of the Drugs & Cosmetic Rules, 1945 for importing the drugs (investigational products, comparators, placebo, etc.). The application should give a detailed calculation of the quantity of drugs required for the study and from which country; these drugs are to be imported. The DCGI issues Test Licence (popularly known as T Licence) in Form 11 of the Drugs and Cosmetic Rules for the import of drugs. Since this application is made concurrently, the 'T Licence' is obtained along with the permission for the clinical trial. Hence, it is not allowed to import the drugs without DCGI approval and T Licence. The validity of the T Licence is for a period of 1 year.

Export of Biological Samples: The Formalities

Sponsor/its representative intending to export human biological specimens e.g., tissues, blood, etc. to destinations out of India for test purposes, should apply for export permission from the Director General of Foreign Trade (DGFT), India. The application should be made using the Form specified in DGFT policy and procedure for grant of export licence for items mentioned as restricted for exports in schedule ii of ITC (HS) classifications of export and imports items. The blood and blood products are classified as restricted item for exports. The Sponsor/its representative should have the Importer Exporter Code Number (IEC) which needs to be mentioned in the application.

Besides this, the application shall provide the details of the laboratory, where the blood / plasma sample is to be exported, the tests and procedures to be performed with the sample and the quantity of blood and number of samples to be collected from each subject and the number of shipments to be sent. A declaration from the central laboratory shall also be submitted along with the application stating that the blood/plasma samples collected from India will not be misused for genetic purposes or otherwise. This application can be submitted concurrently, but the export permission for the same will be obtained from DGFT office, only after submitting the 'No objection certificate and/or clinical trial permission from the DCGI'. This process may take 1–2 weeks after receiving the clinical trial permission.

However, there is a proposal with the DCGI to create a system of single window clearance for clinical trial permission, import permission/test licence for import of study drugs and export permission for human biological samples. Although there is a single window mechanism in place for the clinical trial permission and import of investigational products through the DCGI's office, the export permission is still to be obtained from DGFT's office. Maybe over time, the Government of India will synchronise the same to facilitate the clinical trial approval process.

Protection of Intellectual Property and Patents

In January 2005, Indian government has issued an Ordinance amending the Patent Act, 1970, which is compliant to Trade Related Intellectual Property Rights (TRIPS) under the World Trade Organization (WTO) mandated product patent regime. As a signatory to TRIPS and WTO, India has moved from an era of process patent to product patent regime. This commitment of Government has changed the business environment, increased R&D initiative by both local and global companies and a lot of foreign investment by the global companies.

India has positioned herself as a global R&D and manufacturing hub, which attracts global investment because of lower cost manufacturing supported by adequate regulatory protection of intellectual property. Most of the success of Indian companies could be attributable to the number of patents filed with USFDA in recent years. India has filed a total of 126 DMFs with USFDA, accounting for 20 per cent of all drugs coming into the US market, higher than Spain, Italy, Israel, and China. Of the 108 Abbreviated New Drug Applications (ANDA) pending approval from the USFDA in February 2004, as many as 52 were patent challenges and nearly half of these were for first to file (180 days market exclusivity).

The large success of Indian pharmacos in the generics has established their capability in the manufacturing and process chemistry business. Hence, many global pharmaceutical companies have also decided to source their bulk requirements from India and outsource their manufacturing to local companies.

Hence, by embracing intellectual property and amending the patent Act to accommodate product patent rather than process patent, India has already started witnessing significant growth in foreign direct investment and increased R&D. The enforcement of this robust patent system with patent protection is a positive step for all the pharmaceutical multinational companies (MNCs) to tap the Indian market without fear of their products being copied.

Indian Experience of Trials and Audit

India has witnessed global multicentric clinical trials in last 8–10 years. Most of these studies are conducted by global companies like Pfizer, Eli Lilly, GSK, Novartis, Novo Nordisk, Aventis, Quintiles, etc. Although, there are not many USFDA audits or regulatory inspections being carried out in India to substantiate the quality of data, there are several mock audits and quality assurance audits carried out by the sponsors in each of these global studies. The reports of the quality assurance auditors and/or the third party independent auditors are quite positive about the data quality, integrity and accuracy.[4–7]

India: Cost Advantage

There are several estimates of cost advantage (ranging from 40–60%) of doing trials in India vis-à-vis western countries. Although, cost is one of the important deciding parameters, it is always linked with the quality of services while assessing a project in a particular territory.

However, the major indirect cost advantage is the fast recruitment, i.e. 4–5 times higher than the rate of recruitment in USA and Europe in any therapeutic area leading to lots of savings in time and money. The cost of treatment including the tests and procedures may be 40–50% less than the comparative cost in USA and Europe. Similarly, the cost of skilled labor in India is very low in comparison. A clinical trial monitor typically earns approximately 10–15% of his USA/European counterpart.

While it is mostly assured that there will be a lot of saving in per patient cost because of first recruitment and low cost of test and procedure, the charge out rates of the service providers may not reduce in the same proportion. For example, if the sponsor wishes to avail the services of a global service provider like World Courier, who are specialized in certain services, the cost of the service in India may be low, but may not be 40–50% less in comparison to western countries. Similarly, the CRO fees are dependent on many factors including the cost of the skilled employees and the other overheads of creating and maintaining a global standard infrastructure like broad band connectivity, access control, fire and smoke alarm and detectors, adequate working space, ambient working environment for monitors, etc. in a prime location with proper connectivity, which involve a lot of cost. And again there are important variants like increased air travel cost and more travel time as most of the sites are geographically spread in diverse locations. But overall, a lot of cost savings can be generated.

Efficacy Results: Indian *vs.* Caucasian Population

India has an ethnically mixed population. Several studies in the past have proven that efficacy results in Indian population are similar to those of the Caucasian population but were significantly different from those of the Japanese/Chinese population. But trials in the past also have proven otherwise in some therapeutic areas. There could be difference in dosage level where the requirement for an average Indian patient may be lower in comparison to the individual from a developed country.

Social Security/Health Insurance Policy

In India, there is no social security or public healthcare insurance for all. Public spending on healthcare is low compared to the developed countries. According to some estimates, only 3% of India's population is covered under some form of voluntary health insurance. Today, the middle-class segment is increasing and many of them are now choosing to purchase health insurance from private/public insurance companies with either full or partial coverage. In this scenario, clinical trial participation, follow up, compliance is better in India as the patients participating in a clinical trial are getting the benefit of medication and treatment, which otherwise is generally not covered under the health insurance system of the country.

Other Concerns

Besides this, there are many other global concerns which are administrative in nature and can be sorted out through a well-trained and dedicated project management system. For example, a complaint of delay in custom clearance by many can be sorted out through proper knowledge of import documentation, pre-approval of consignment (if the consignment is temperature sensitive), choosing a proper custom clearing agent, etc. The other issues which cause concern for many pharmaceutical sponsors are whether to market the drug in India and if so, at what price. Few other concerns which are noteworthy to Indian context are, illiteracy and translation of consent forms and patient information sheet, whether to continue the trial medications to clinical trial patients even after study is over, etc.

CONCLUSION

India can accommodate the contract research business expansions because of the availability of huge **talent pool** of Investigators and clinical research professionals. The growth in pharmaceutical and biotech manufacturing, and contract research supported by IT skills has also led to promising outsourcing business in various other segments including clinical trial data management, statistical analysis. This is so far a win-win situation and the success depends on sustainability with continued maintenance of good quality and no complacency.

REFERENCES

1. Sahoo U (2005). Bhatt A 2010 - Indian Clinical Research Odyssey–Pharmabiz, February, 26, 2004, www.pharmabiz.com
2. Schedule Y, Amended Version 2005 http://www.cdsco.nic.in/html/Schedule-Y%20(Amended%20Version-2005)%20original.htm
3. GCP for clinical research in India http://www.cdsco.nic.in/html/GCP.htm
4. Sahoo U (2005). Clinical Research Careers–Looking up. Monitor. October 2005. p37-42. http://www.acrpnet.org/resources/monitor/membersonly/october05/sahoo.pdf
5. Sahoo U (2005). Clinical Trial Data Management Outsourcing India; A Review of Cost and Competition. Eye for Pharma, http://www.eyeforpharma.com/briefing/India2.pdf#search='data%20management%20sahoo'
6. Sen Falguni (2005), Conducting Clinical Trials: Is There An India Advantage, ACRP Monitor, December, 2005, http://www.acrpnet.org/resources/monitor
7. Sahoo U (2005). Laboratories and Clinical Trial in India–ACRP Monitor, Summer 2004. http://www.acrpnet.org/resources/monitor/archive/index.html

Chapter 4

Basics of Bioanalytical Method Development for Isotretinoin using LC-MS/MS

.Nageshwar Rao Thudi
T.K. Pal

BASICS OF BIOANALYTICAL METHOD DEVELOPMENT

Introduction to Method Development

Bioanalytics is the application of analytical technique to determine drug or metabolite concentrations in biological matrix samples mostly in plasma, serum or urine samples related to Bioavailability and Bioequivalence studies. It plays a key role throughout the drug development from discovery to drug approval.

The field of bioanalytics covers a wide cross-section of modern analytical techniques and advanced equipments. It is very important to decide whether we require estimating only analyte(s) or metabolite(s) or both before starting method development.

CRITICAL STEPS INVOLVED

Planning

That includes literature search, molecular structure, basic chemistry, selection of instrument and technique, availability of instruments, columns, chemicals, trained analysts and finally discussions.

A. Literature search

That includes internet, journals and availability of methods for structurally similar compounds.

B. Chemical structure and basic chemistry

Acids: carboxyl, phenolic, sulfonic, sulfonamide, imide (-CO-NH-CO-), β-carbonyl group (-CO-CHR-CO-), ammonium salts, bases- NH_2, -NHR, -NR$_2$, hydroxyl groups, neutral- ketones, aldehydes, esters, ethers, hydrocarbons, nitriles, alkyl halides, alcohols, amides.

The important point to be remembered when dealing with carboxylic acid group compounds is that it should loose CO_2 (–44 daltons) in negative mode scanning and acidic compounds ionize much better in negative mode as compared to positive mode unless until it is suppressed by mobile phase buffers like TFA, sulfonic acids. (Addition of acid will suppress negative ion signal intensity since weakly acidic compounds will not be de-protonated in an acidic solution).

C. Selection of ionization source

Atmospheric pressure ionization (API) for low molecular weight and easily ionizable molecules.

Atmospheric pressure chemical ionization (APCI) for neutral and high molecular weight molecules (usually above 500 daltons).

D. Selection of mobile phase buffer

It is recommended that all solvents used in HPLC or LC/MS are degassed. Degassing may be achieved by sonication or vacuum filtration using 0.22 micron membrane filter.

(Highly) recommended solvents LC-MS/MS or HPLC: Water, acetonitrile and methanol and suitable solvents (but used infrequently): Ethanol and 2-propanol (Table 4.1).

During method development it is advised not to mix the buffer and solvent together in large proportions unless until binary or quaternary HPLC pumps are not available to avoid wastage of the solvent.

Modifiers, buffers, etc.

For HPLC: Sodium acetate, sodium bicarbonate, potassium dihydrogen phosphate, potassium ortho-phosphate, ammonium acetate, pentane, butane, heptane, sulfonic acids, etc.

For LC-MS/MS: Basic compounds will usually show an enhanced signal by lowering the pH of the mobile phase. Strong, volatile acids such as formic (and/or acetic) are recommended. Adding 0.1 to 1.0% is usually sufficient to enhance MS ionization but LC requirements may require a higher concentration. Addition of acid will suppress *negative ion* signal intensity since weakly acidic compounds will not be de-protonated in an acidic solution.

Ammonium formate or acetate is suitable mobile phase buffers for use in LC/MS. Usually, 2–10 mM concentration is adequate but concentrations as high as 50 mM can be used. Ammonium acetate may be used to replace phosphate buffers, which *are not recommended for LC/MS*.

Ammonium adducts will frequently be observed in (+) ion operation and formate or acetate adducts will be observed in (–) ion operation.

Ammonium hydroxide may also be used for LC/MS if the pH of the mobile phase needs to be reduced. All of the ammonium buffers may enhance sensitivity of weakly acidic compounds undergoing (–) ion analysis.

Non-recommended agents

Any non-volatile salts. These will crystallize during droplet desolvation and will *plug the orifice*, the Ion Spray needle and fused silica tubing. *Phosphate buffers are not recommended*.

Ion pairing agents should **not** be used for Ion Spray LC/MS.

Detergents and surfactants should be avoided. These are extremely sensitive to Ion Spray analysis and consequently will suppress the ionization of other compounds.

Inorganic acids such as H_2SO_4 and H_3PO_4 should be avoided along as well as HCl since all of these will suppress ionization of target compounds.

Other LC/MS solvents reported in the literature

Triethlyamine (TEA) has been used but it may suppress the ionization of less basic compounds in (+) ion operation (and it gives an intense ion at m/z 102). It may be used in (−) ion mode to enhance ionization of other compounds.

Tetrahydrofuran (THF) has been used as an additive in LC/MS. High concentrations of THF should be used *with extreme caution* in APCI operation with the heated nebulizer due to flammability. Air should **not** be used for the nebulizer or auxiliary gas in APCI operation. Peek tubing should be avoided when using THF.

Normal phase solvents

Dichloromethane, toluene and hexane have been used in normal phase LC/MS.

Solvents properties for Mobile Phase (HPLC/ LC MS)

Table 4.1: UV cutoff of common solvents

Solvent	UV Cutoff	Solvent	UV Cutoff
Water	180	Heptane	197
Methanol	205	Cyclohexane	200
N-Propanol	205	Carbon tetrachloride	265
Acetonitrile	190	Chloroform	245
THF	225	Benzene	280
Acetone	330	Toluene	285
Methyl acetate	260	Methylene chloride	232
Ethyl acetate	260	Tetrachloroethylene	280
Nitromethane	380	1, 2-Dichloroethane	225

E. Ionization constant (pKa)

For pH adjustment and also for ionization
　　Percent ionization = Rule of nine

If　pH − pka = 1 then 90% (1 nine)
　　pH − pka = 2 then 99% (2 nines)
　　pH − pka = 3 then 99.9% (3 nines)

F. Flexibility for stable labeled internal standards

For ring deuteration of benzene, fast avenues could be the Griess reaction, namely reduction of benzenediazonium salts in deuterated ethanol: (perhaps better with higher alcohol homologs).

$$PhN_3+ Cl^- + R{-}OD \longrightarrow Ph{-}D + Ph{-}OR$$

Conditions may be chosen to favor deuteration, although a final distillation may be required to separate the ether.

An alternative is desulfonation of aromatic sulfonic acids with hot deuterium oxide:

$$Ph{-}SO_3D + D_2O \longrightarrow Ph{-}D + D_2SO_4$$

Both processes are applicable to aromatics other than benzene.

For deuteration at the alpha position of toluene, catalytic deuterolysis of benzyl ether can be affected:

$$PhCH_2-OR + D_2 \longrightarrow PhCH_2-D + RO-D$$

Deuteration of alkyl aromatics at farther removed positions may be carried out via the Grignard reaction:

$$R\ Br + Mg \longrightarrow R-MgBr$$

$$R-MgBr + D_2O \longrightarrow R-D + DO-MgBr$$

G. Selection of instrument/technique

Depending upon availability, sensitivity requirement, timeliness, volatility, stability and recovery HPLC (UV, ECD, and fluorescence), GC MS MS, LC MS MS and immunoassays can be selected.

H. Selection of HPLC column

Depending upon the nature of the analytes reverse phase or normal phase columns for HPLC can be selected. It is very important that these columns should be purchased from authorized suppliers only and the column performance should be done as per the manufacturer certificate or as per the SOP of the lab.

Some of the examples for reverse phase columns are C18, C8, C4, etc. and for normal phase columns are CN, amino, silica, etc. (Table 4.2).

Carbon load (C4, C8, and C18), diameter and flow rate adjustment depending upon the diameter place a key role in separation, selectivity and sensitivity of a method.

Column id and flow rate

4.6 mm	1.0 ml/min
2.1 mm	0.2 ml/min
1.0 mm	0.05 ml/min

The effect of column id on sensitivity

Column id relative sensitivity

4.6 mm	–
3.0 mm	2.3
2.1 mm	4.8
1.0 mm	21 times

As the column internal diameter decreases, the volume of the chromatographic peaks decreases, concentrating the sample and increasing sensitivity. If the same amount of sample is injected, a column with an id of 2.1 mm will give about 5 fold the sensitivity of a column with an id of 4.6 mm.

Table 4.2: The commonly used column dimensions for different instruments

S.No.	Instrument	Length (mm)	Width (mm)	Particle Size (µ)	Plates (per meter)
1	HPLC	150 to 300	4 to 4.6	5 to 10	50,000
2	LC MS MS	50 to 75	2 to 4.6	3	
3	GC	30 meters	0.25	0.25	3000 (capillary)

I. Estimation of active drug, metabolite (or both) when?

Any decision to use metabolite data in bioequivalence studies, however, must be made prior to avoiding introduction of bias arising from selective post hoc manipulation of the raw data; and to facilitate the design of blood sampling schedules based on prior information about the tmax of the selected analyte.

Measurement of a metabolite may be preferred when parent drug levels are too low to allow reliable analytical measurement in blood, plasma, or serum for an adequate length of time. FDA recommends that the metabolite data obtained from these studies be subjected to a confidence interval approach for BE demonstration.

If there is a clinical concern related to efficacy or safety for the parent drug, FDA also recommend that sponsors and/or applicants contact the appropriate review division to determine whether the parent drug should be measured and analyzed statistically.

A metabolite may be formed as a result of gut wall or other presystemic metabolism.

If the metabolite contributes meaningfully to safety and/or efficacy, FDA also recommends that the metabolite and the parent drug be measured. When the relative activity of the metabolite is low and does not contribute meaningfully to safety and/or efficacy, it does not have to be measured. FDA recommends that the parent drug measured in these BE studies be analyzed using a confidence interval approach. The metabolite data can be used to provide supportive evidence of comparable therapeutic outcome.

Example: Prodrugs like Nabumetone (6-MNA), Valgnacyclovir (Gancyclovir) and sometimes both active moiety as well as metabolite (venlafaxine and des acetyl venlafaxine: Quinapril and Quinaprilat) for safety and efficacy. It is all depends on the country which we are submitting or planning to release the drug.

J. LOQ and calibration curve requirements

Ideal bioanalytical method has to detect the analyte conc. upto 3 half life's and is at least 0.05 X Cmax.

UOQ can be X*Cmax, X can be 1, 2, 3, 4, depending on the magnitude of variability on Cmax (influencing factors such as induction, inhibition, air, light and all physical and mythological elements).

K. Biological matrix (whole blood, plasma, serum, urine, etc.)

When the analyte drug is extensively bounded to red blood cells, the bioanalytical method has to be developed using whole blood of healthy volunteers (not in a plasma – blood/plasma ratio is ~6:1).

When repeated blood samples from certain patient populations, for example very young, pediatric patients the apparent volume of distribution may be so large that plasma concentrations are too small to measure it may be important to determine the role of metabolism in the elimination of a drug. Analysis of urine data for unchanged drug and metabolite concentrations is essential to the quantitative study of drug metabolism.

Urinary excretion of the unchanged drug is directly proportional to the plasma concentration of total drug. Thus, the total quantity of drug excreted in the urine is a reflection of the quantity of drug absorbed from the gastrointestinal tract.

This technique of studying bioavailability is most useful for those drugs that are not extensively metabolized prior to urinary elimination. As a rule of thumb, determination of bioavailability using urinary excretion data should be conducted only if at least 20% of a dose is excreted unchanged in the urine after an IV dose.

Other conditions which must be met for this method to give valid results include:

(*a*) The fraction of drug entering the bloodstream and being excreted intact by the kidneys must remain constant.

(*b*) Collection of the urine has to continue until all the drug has been completely excreted (five times the half-life 1).

IMPLEMENTATION

Optimization of detection and chromatography condition, establishment of extraction technique for selectivity, sensitivity, etc. and finally stability study.

Extraction and Recovery

Precipitation, liquid-liquid extraction, solid phase extraction and immunoassays, etc.

Extraction - using pH/pKa partitioning or lipid/aqueous solubility differences extraction can be used to remove unwanted interfering compounds or to concentrate the compound(s) of interest. The use of various organic solvents of differing polarity and/or aqueous buffers can provide excellent resolution based on the solubility of the free compounds of interest and/or their salt forms. Extraction may be used to remove lipophilic interfering compounds or to remove the desirable compounds into a cleaner environment.

Characteristics of Solvents

Polarity	Solvent	Miscible in Water?
Nonpolar		
	Hexane	No
	Isooctane	No
	Carbon tetrachloride	No
	Chloroform	No
	Methylene chloride	No
	Tetrahydrofuran	Yes
	Diethyl ether	No
	Ethyl acetate	Poorly
	Acetone	Yes
	Acetonitrile	Yes
	Isopropanol	Yes
	Methanol	Yes
	Water	Yes
Polar	Acetic acid	Yes

INTRODUCTION AND PHARMACOKINETICS OF ISOTRETINOIN

Introduction

Isotretinoin; 13-cis retinoic acid: (2Z, 4E, 6E, 8E)-3, 7-dimethyl-9-(2,6,6-trimethylcyclohexen-1-yl) nona-2,4,6,8-tetraenoic acid. It has a molecular formula and weight of $C_{20}H_{28}O_2$ and 300.42 respectively. (Fig. 4.1)

Isotretinoin is a retinoid, which when administered in pharmacologic dosages of 0.5 to 1.0 mg/kg/day inhibits sebaceous gland function and keratinization. The exact mechanism of action is unknown.

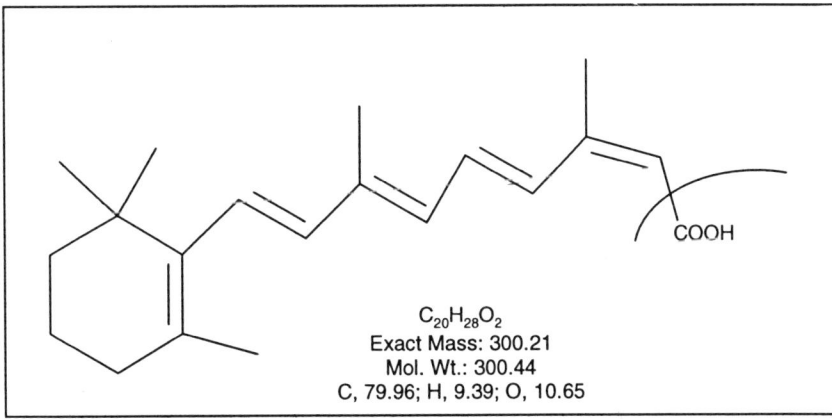

Fig. 4.1. Molecular structure of isotretinoin and its possible fragmentation

Pharmacokinetics of Isotretinoin

Absorption

Peak plasma concentrations (C_{max}) of approximately 200–300 ng/ml have been achieved in healthy volunteers three to four hours (t_{max}) after administration of 40 mg isotretinoin. Taking isotretinoin with food increases bioavailability up to twofold relative to fasting conditions, probably as a result of easier absorption of this highly lipophilic medication. Furthermore, there is an overall decrease in fluctuations in systemic availability when isotretinoin is ingested with food.

Distribution

Isotretinoin is more than 99.9% bound to plasma proteins, primarily albumin.

Metabolism

Following oral administration of isotretinoin, at least three metabolites have been identified in human plasma: 4-*oxo*-isotretinoin, retinoic acid (tretinoin), (Fig. 4.2) and 4-*oxo*-retinoic acid (4-*oxo*-tretinoin).

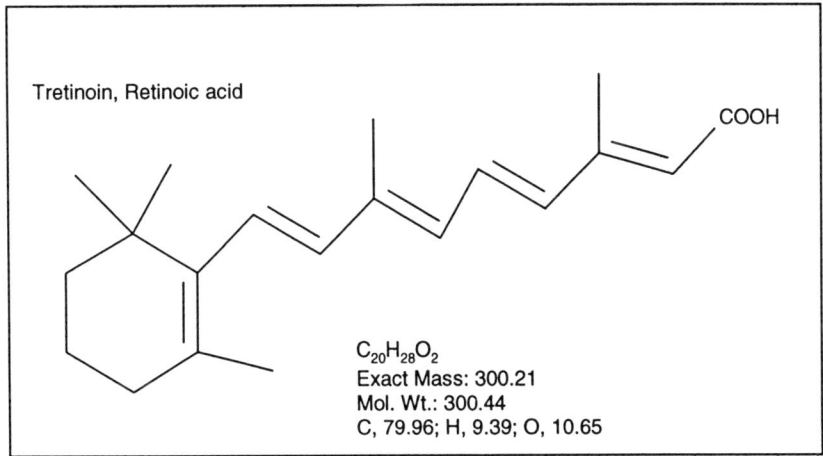

Fig. 4.2. Molecular structure of tretinoin

Retinoic acid and 13-*cis*-retinoic acid are geometric isomers and show reversible interconversion. The administration of one isomer will give rise to the other. Isotretinoin is also irreversibly oxidized to 4-*oxo*-isotretinoin, which forms its geometric isomer 4-*oxo*-tretinoin (Fig. 4.3).

After a single 80 mg oral dose of Accutane to 74 healthy adult subjects, concurrent administration of food increased the extent of formation of all metabolites in plasma when compared to the extent of formation under fasted conditions.

All of these metabolites possess retinoid activity that is in some in vitro models more than that of the parent isotretinoin. However, the clinical significance of these models is unknown. After multiple oral dose administration of isotretinoin to adult cystic acne patients, the exposure of patients to 4-*oxo*-isotretinoin at steadystate under fasted and fed conditions was approximately 3.4 times higher than that of isotretinoin.

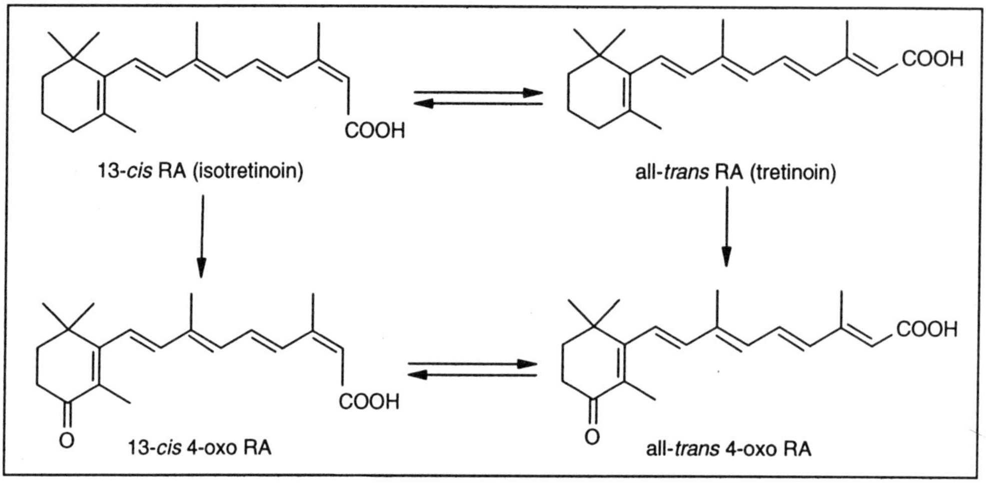

Fig. 4.3. Isotretinoin and metabolites

In vitro studies indicate that the primary P450 isoforms involved in isotretinoin metabolism are 2C8, 2C9, 3A4, and 2B6. Isotretinoin and its metabolites are further metabolized into conjugates, which are then excreted in urine and feces.

Elimination

Following oral administration of an 80 mg dose of ^{14}C-isotretinoin as a liquid suspension, ^{14}C-activity in blood declined with a half-life of 90 hours. The metabolites of isotretinoin and any conjugates are ultimately excreted in the feces and urine in relatively equal amounts (total of 65% to 83%). After a single 80 mg oral dose of Accutane to 74 healthy adult subjects under fed conditions, the mean SD elimination half-lives ($t_{1/2}$) of isotretinoin and 4-*oxo*-isotretinoin were 21.0, 8.2 hours and 24.0, 5.3 hours, respectively. After both single and multiple doses, the observed accumulation ratios of isotretinoin ranged from 0.90 to 5.43 in patients with cystic acne.

Protocol for Method Development of Isotretinoin

Planning

Since both isotretinoin and tretinoin metabolites are having the same molecular weight and MRM transition, these have to be separated chromatographically and then quantified using MRM transition method of mass spectrometer. This method was developed based on the chemical structure, literature, pKa and also by using statistical software, etc.

Chromatographic separation and estimation by LC-MS/MS is the best idea but expensive technique for this kind of methods. But due to better sensitivity, specificity and faster analysis, LC-MS/MS method is having advantage over 25 to 30 minutes HPLC methods.

Mobile phase

Since LC-MS/MS requires to use volatile buffers, following buffers with different concentrations and with various solvents have been tried:

2 to 10 mM Ammonium acetate (pH 10.4 to 10.6): acetonitrile (45:55 to 30:70) **or** 2 to 10 mM ammonium acetate (pH 10.4 to 10.6): acetonitrile: methanol (40:30:30 to 30:35:35) **or** 2 to 10 mM ammonium acetate (pH 10.4 to 10.6): methanol (45:55 to 30:70)

HPLC column: C18; 150, 100, 50 mm × 4.6 mm

Flow rate: 0.6 to 1.2 mL/min

Extraction procedure: To 0.5 to 0.8 mL plasma add 0.2 to 0.3 mL buffer (pH around 6.0) vortex, and add 5 to 7 mL ter. butyl methyl ether or hexane or hexane: iso-amyl alcohol (98:2), shake for 15 minutes on horizontal shaker, then centrifuge it for 8 to 10 minutes at 2500 RPM and flash freeze the samples using acetone and dry ice bath. Separate the organic layer and dry it under steam of nitrogen gas at 40°C and recon in 150 to 200 µL mobile phase.

Injection volume: Various injection volumes from 10 to 50 µL.

LOQ required: 1.00 to 1.50 ng/mL.

Internal standards planned: Since acitretin is structurally similar to isotretinoin, it is proposed as internal standard and please refer to the structure below (Fig. 4.4).

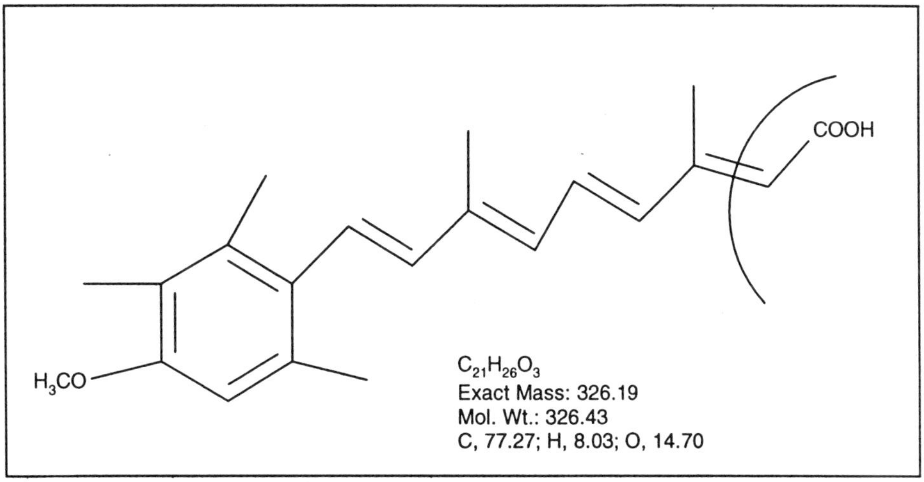

$C_{21}H_{26}O_3$
Exact Mass: 326.19
Mol. Wt.: 326.43
C, 77.27; H, 8.03; O, 14.70

Fig. 4.4. Molecular structure with possible fragmentation of acitretin

Schimadzu LC10 or HP1100 series HPLC system along with API 2000 or 3000 mass spectrometer is required to achieve the desired sensitivity.

Table 4.3: Expected (theoretical) m/z in negative and positive mode

	$(M-H)^-$	$(M+H)^+$
Isotretinoin/ Tretinoin	299.2	301.2
Acetritin	325.2	327.2

Implementation

Standard solution preparation

Upon request AAI Pharma, USA has supplied isotretinoin, tretinoin and acetritin compounds.

1 mg/mL stock solutions were prepared using methanol as a diluent for all three compounds. Further dilutions were made in methanol: water (60:40).

Mass confirmation (Q1 MS method)

Initially for the confirmation of mass, solution of 500 ng/mL was prepared individually for all three compounds and injected continuously using syringe pump method at the rate of 10 µL/min. Mass was scanned from 100 to 650 m/z using product ion scan in both negative and positive mode. Both negative and positive ionizations were checked in API (electro spray ionization) source (Table 4.3).

Mass optimization (MS/MS method)

For better optimization and to prevent the effect on ionization by each other, all three compounds were diluted up to 100 ng/mL in single solution. Using this solution all compound parameters were optimized individually for each compound (Table 4.4).

Table 4.4: Compound (MS/MS) parameters

S.No.	Compound	DP	FP	CE
1	Isotretinoin/ Tretinoin	35	−250	−20
2	Acitritin	25	−200	−25

Fragmentation and mass spectra of isotretinoin

Initially the Q1 MS optimization was done in API ionization source in both positive and negative mode and negative (−) polarity (M-H) was selected based on enough sensitivity, selectivity (less signal to noise ratio) and to avoid excessive fragmentation.

For the parent-product scans used for all three compounds please refer to MRM transition in Table 4.5.

Table 4.5: Final MRM transition ions

S.No.	Analyte/ ISTD	MRM transition
1.	Isotretinoin/ tretinoin	299.3/ 255.1
2.	Acetritin	325.3/ 266.3

HPLC-MS/MS conditions

After finalization of MS and MRM conditions (Table 4.6) the aqueous mixture was injected without any column to finalize the temperature and gases of the source. Then the sample was injected using different columns of different manufactures (as discussed in planning section) and finally all three compounds were well separated from one another (please see the chromatogram of reference solution under method validation section) on Nova pack C18 100 × 4.6 mm at 0.9 ml/min using 10 mM Ammonium acetate (pH 10.5): Methanol at 48:52 proportions. 1:3 split was used before turbo ion spray source and after HPLC column to avoid excess solvent pumping into the source.

Table 4.6: Final MRM conditions for isotretinoin

Scan Type: MRM	Polarity: Negative
Ion Source: Turbo Spray	Resolution Q1: Low
Resolution Q3: High	Step Size: 0.00 amu.
Dwell Time: 150 msec.	Nebulizer Gas : 9.00 at 60 psi
Curtain Gas: 12.00 at 60 psi	Ion Spray Voltage (IS): −4500
Temperature: 425°C	CAD Gas: 5.00
Entrance Potential (EP): −8.00	Collision Cell Exit Potential (CXP): 15

Results and Discussion of Method Validation of Isotretinoin using LC-MS/MS.

After developing above MRM method (Tables 5.0 and 6.0) in LC-MS/MS a trial batch containing a calibration curve and quality control checks was tested before starting a complete method validation.

This bioanalytical method was validated for following parameters (1) selectivity, (2) sensitivity, (3) matrix effect, (4) precision (repeatability), (5) accuracy, (6) recovery, (7) linearity, (8) stability [In-injector (or) post-processing, bench top, freeze-thaw, stock solution short-term and long-term, matrix samples long-term and dilution integrity].

Reference Solution of Isotretinoin Method

A solution containing analyte(s) and ISTD(s) equivalent to unextracted high quality control (HQC) concentration was extracted and injected as a reference solution and representative chromatogram for the same can be seen in Fig. 4.5.

Selectivity for Isotretinoin

Human EDTA plasma from six different donors was collected under controlled time conditions, food ingestion and other important factors as to that of isotretinoin study. Above plasma samples were extracted using the method outlined in extraction procedure and all donors were free of significant interference at the retention of the isotretinoin and its internal standard acitritin. A representative chromatogram for the same can be seen in Fig. 4.6.

Limit of Quantification (LLOQ or Sensitivity) for Isotretinoin

Isotretinoin peak was well identifiable, precise and accurate at its LLOQ concentration in a single run, please see the representative chromatogram for the same (Fig. 4.7). This method has met all the acceptance criteria as required internationally.

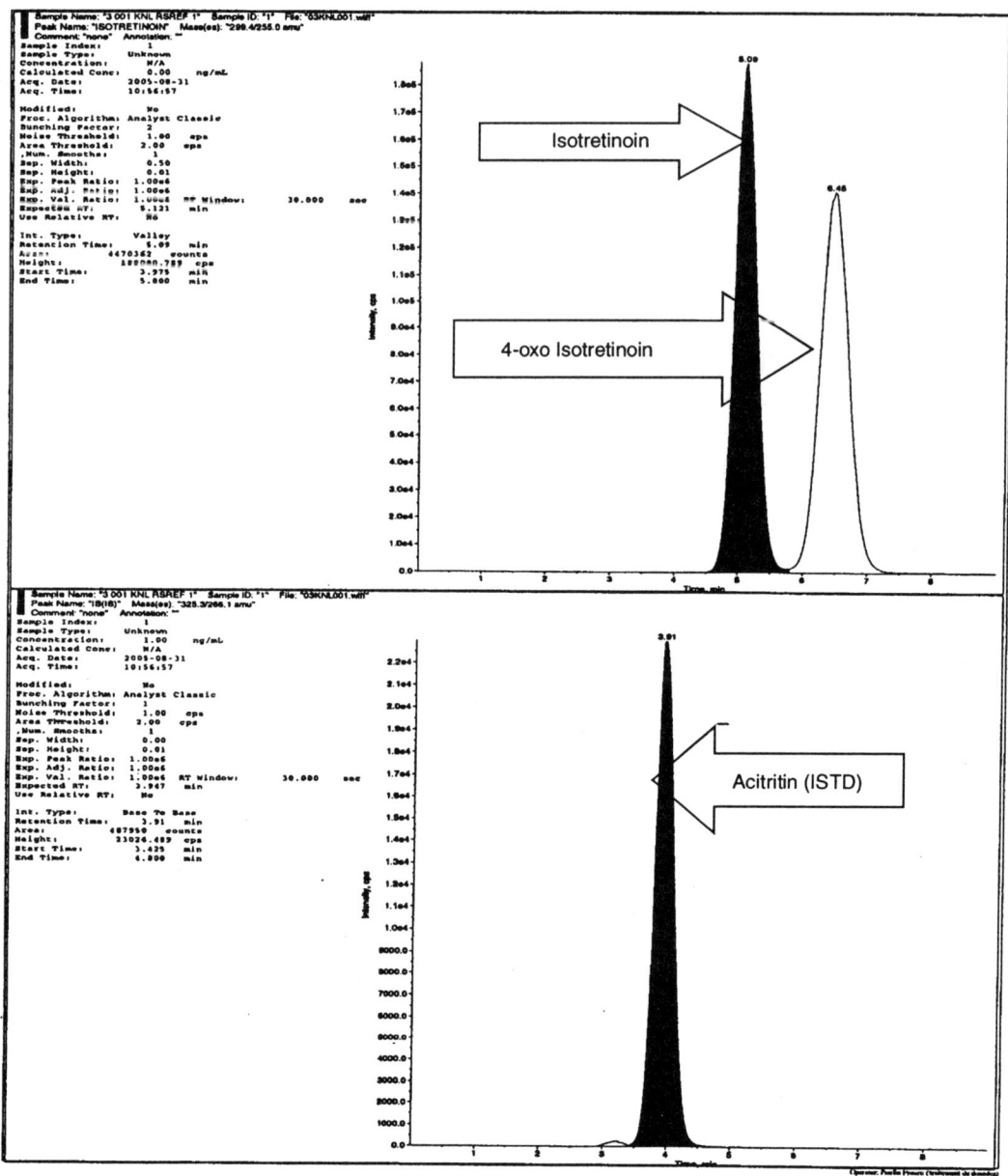

Fig. 4.5. Representative reference chromatogram for isotretinoin

Recovery (Isotretinoin and Internal Standard)

The average recovery was more than 50% for isotretinoin and its internal standard for low, medium and high concentration level and the CV% of the areas for respective concentration and anlyte were within 15%. The results are tabulated in Table 4.7.

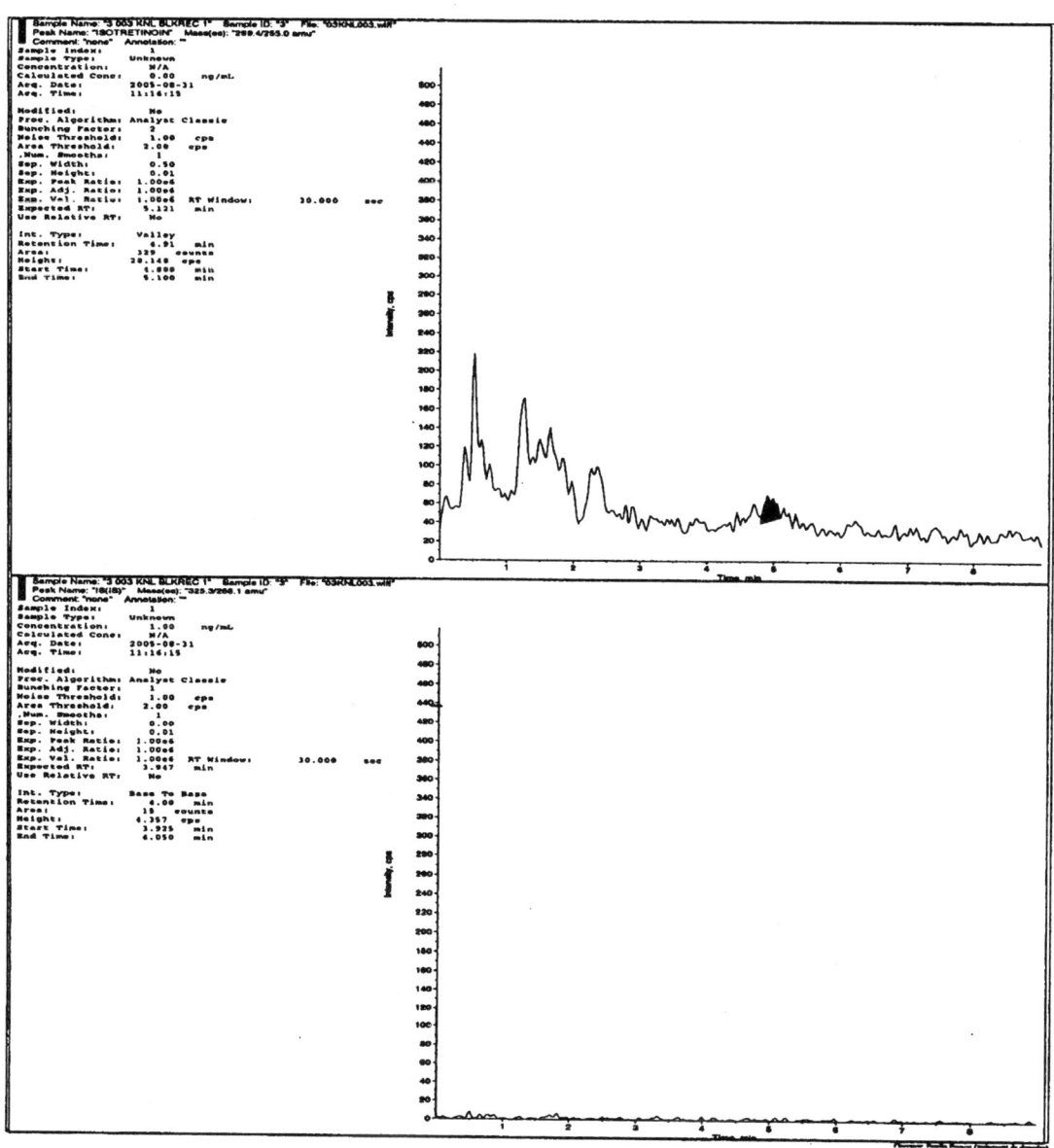

Fig. 4.6. Representative blank chromatogram for isotretinoin

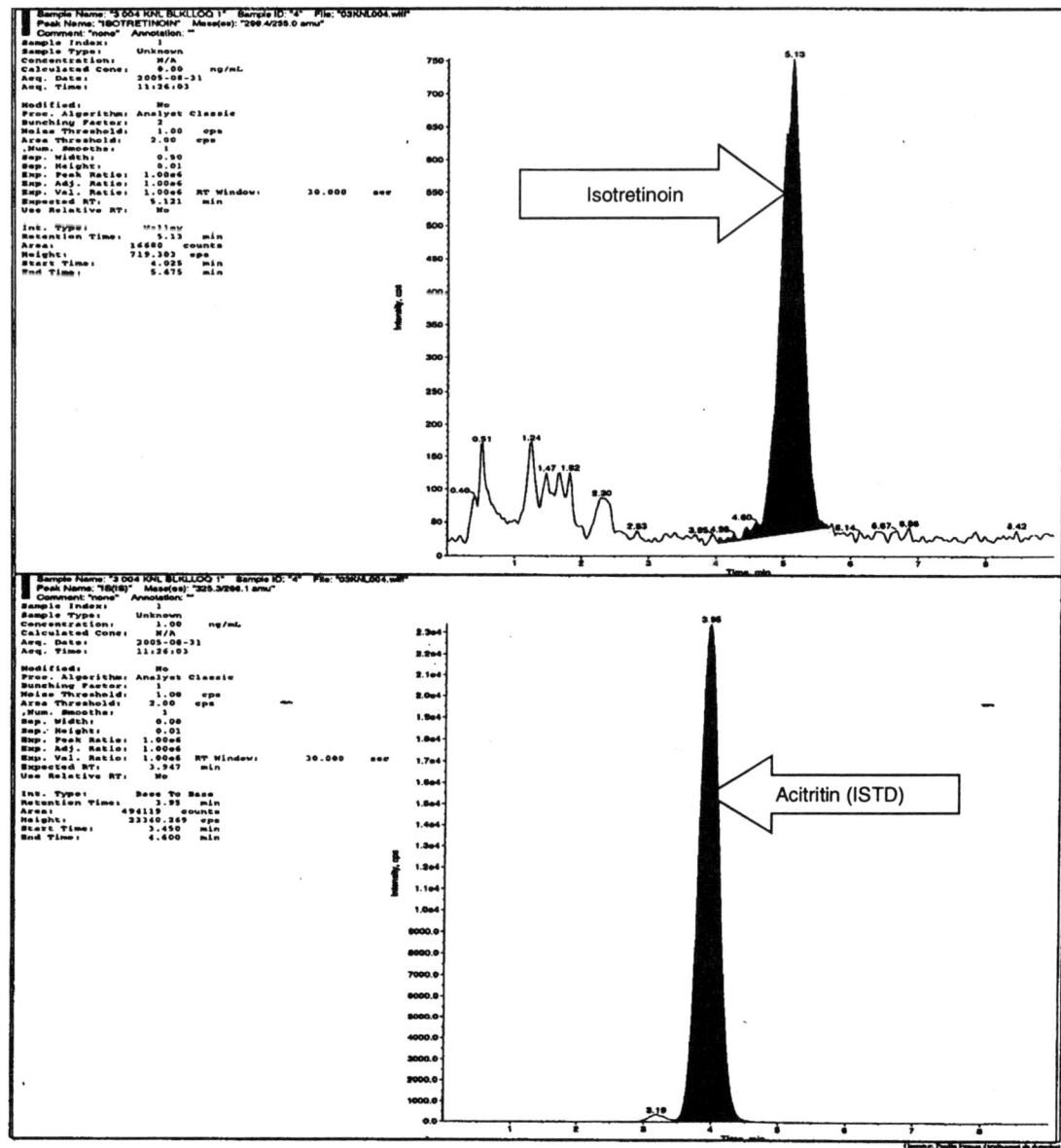

Fig. 4.7. Representative LOQ chromatogram for isotretinoin

Table 4.7. Recovery for analyte (isotretinoin) from plasma

Standard	ID	Unextracted Standard peak area	Extracted matrix Standard peak area	% Recovery
LQC	1	2500	1800	72.00
2.5 (ng/mL)	2	2300	1900	82.61

(Contd.)

(Contd.)

	3	2300	1900	82.61
	4	2300	2000	86.96
	5	2400	2100	87.50
	6	2200	1700	77.27
Mean		2333	1900	81.49
SD (±)		103.2796	141.4214	5.9389
CV%		4.43	7.44	7.29
MQC	1	62000	48000	77.42
75 (ng/mL)	2	65000	42000	64.62
	3	66000	45000	68.18
	4	63000	45000	71.43
	5	66000	44000	66.67
	6	65000	46000	70.77
Mean		64500	45000	69.85
SD (±)		1643.1677	2000.0000	4.4933
CV%		2.55	4.44	6.43
HQC	1	220000	140000	63.64
225 (ng/mL)	2	215000	125000	58.14
	3	215000	142000	66.05
	4	218000	138000	63.30
	5	215000	135000	62.79
	6	216000	132000	61.11
Mean		216500	135333	62.50
SD (±)		2073.6441	6186.0057	2.6661
CV%		0.96	4.57	4.27
			Mean (Avg. of 3 means)	71

Linearity of Isotretinoin

This method proved to be linear for isotretinoin in the range of 1 to 300 ng/mL. All six calibration curves met the acceptance criteria and the r values were more than 0.98. A representative calibration curve can be seen in Fig. 4.8.

Precision and Accuracy of Isotretinoin

Precision and accuracy was determined using fifteen determinations at three concentration levels (excluding blank samples). Both intra and inter day precision and accuracy have been established and CV% was within 15 (Table 4.8). This method has been proved to be precise and accurate in the range of 1 to 300 ng/mL with CV% varies from 6.59 to 10.32 and accuracy from 95.60 to 102.77.

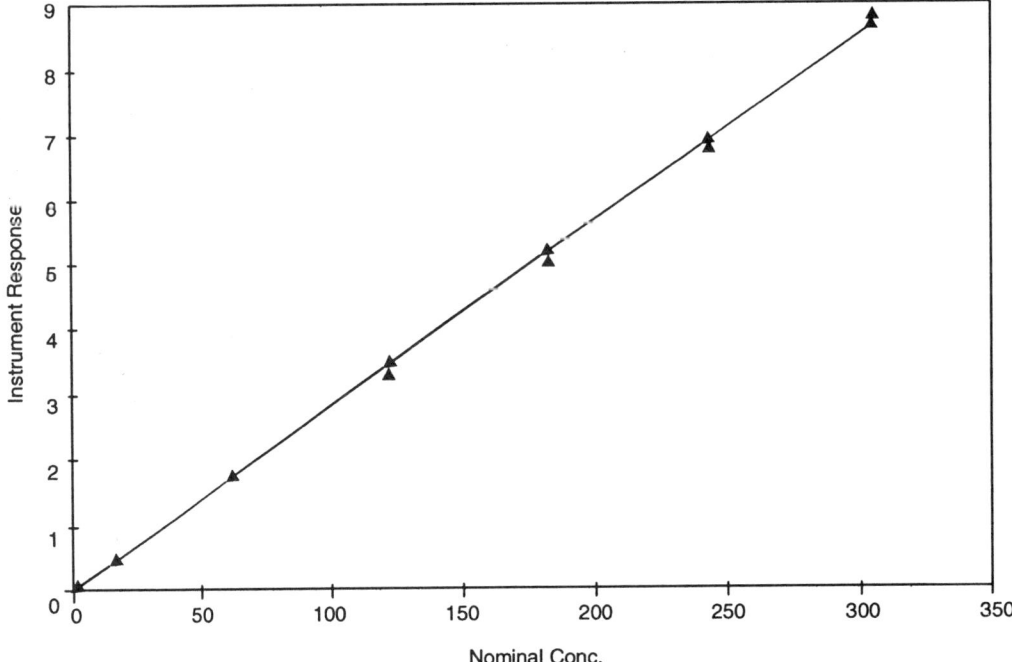

Fig. 4.8. Representative calibration curve for isotretinoin

Table 4.8. Inter-day precision and accuracy for isotretinoin

DAY	ID	LQC (2.5 ng/mL)	MQC (75 ng/mL)	HQC (225 ng/mL)
Day 1-1	1	2.183	71.002	195.234
	2	2.295	83.443	215.991
	3	2.959*	85.246	225.003
	4	2.855	74.103	234.117
	5	3.223*	73.227	196.245
Day 1-2	6	2.097	88.342*	212.743
	7	2.866	69.156	235.751
	8	2.551	65.124	202.523
	9	1.168*	73.245	198.452
	10	2.743	78.446	221.562
Day 2	11	2.474	81.004	231.67
	12	2.771	83.742	224.842
	13	2.826	77.418	210.234
	14	2.653	75.664	222.743
	15	2.516	78.991	199.463
Mean		2.569	76.415	215.105
SD (±)		0.2651	5.8802	14.1822
CV%		10.32	7.70	6.59
% Accuracy		102.77	101.89	95.60

Value outside the acceptable limit

Stabilities of Isotretinoin

Stabilities like Bench Top, freeze thaw, short-term and long-term stock solution and plasma sample stability have been established for isotretinoin at two low and high QC concentration levels and they were within acceptable limit and find the details below and in Fig. 4.9.

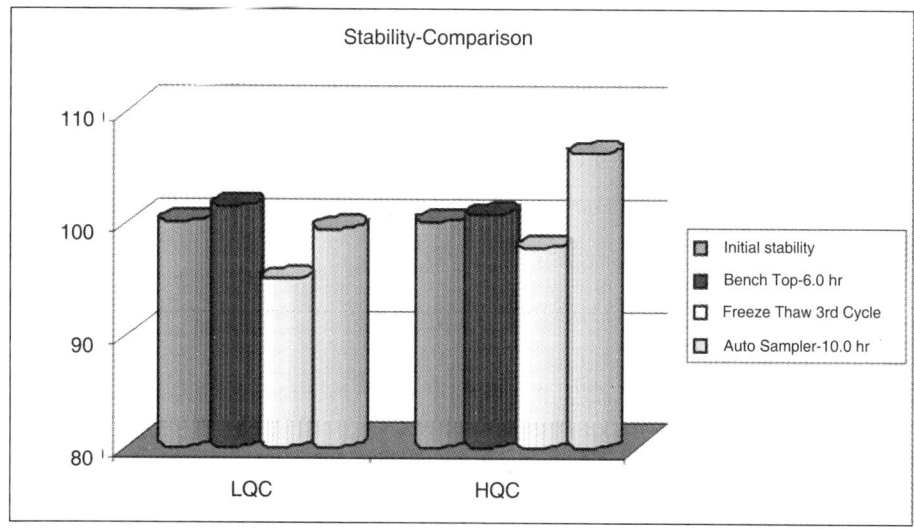

Fig. 4.9. Graphical representation of different stabilities of isotretinoin

This method has been proved to be stable up to 6 hr at room temperature (on bench top), up to 3 freeze thaw cycles at −15°C, up to 10 hrs at 5°C in the auto sampler, hence at least 2 subjects can be extracted at a time and injected continuously.

Stock Solution Stability

Aqueous solution of stocks of isotretinoin, tretinoin and acitritin found to be stable up to 25 days at 4°C.

Plasma Long Term Storage Stability

Isotretinoin spiked plasma samples were found to be stable up to 45 days at −15°C.

Matrix Affect on Isotretinoin

The affect of matrix on the analyte(s) retention time (RT) was studied by spiking and analyzing at low quality concentration (LQC) in six different matrix samples. The back calculated values obtained were within 85 to 115% of actual spiked concentration (Fig. 4.10).

Isotretinoin Method Summary

The above method is found to be linear over the range of 1.0 to 300 ng/mL for isotretinoin. This method is simple, rapid, sensitive, cost-effective, precise and accurate method for pharmacokinetic, bioavailability and bioequivalence studies. This method has no matrix effect and can be used to analyze the samples from wide variety of human subjects. The stock solution can be used without any issues for the minimum period of 25 days. It has minimum met all the stability requirements and can be used for pharmacokinetic and bioequivalence evaluation of any commercially available strengths of isotretinoin.

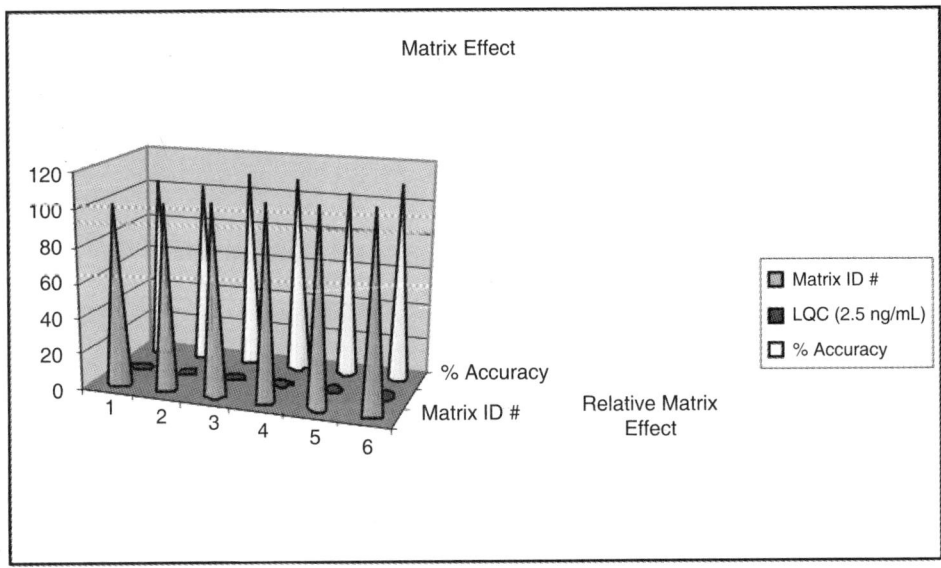

Fig. 4.10. Graphical representation of matrix effect at different concentration levels

REFERENCES

1. Jack Cazes, Raymond P.W. Scott: Chromatography Theory, CRC; 1 edition (March 22, 2002)

2. Raymond P.W. Scott: Liquid Chromatography for the Analyst, CRC; 1 edition (January 17, 1994)

3. James M. Miller: Chromatography: Concepts and Contrasts, Wiley-Interscience; 2 edition (November 29, 2004)

4. Lloyd R. Snyder, Joseph J. Kirkland: Introduction to Modern Liquid Chromatography. 54. Lloyd R. Snyder, Joseph J. Kirkland, Joseph L. Glajch: Practical HPLC Method Development, 2nd Edition.

5. Paul C. Sadek: Troubleshooting HPLC Systems; a Bench Manual, Wiley-Interscience; 1 edition (October 5, 1999)

6. www.chem.csus.edu/forkey/Extraction/Forkeys_extraction.html.

7. Robert E. Ardrey: Liquid Chromatography Mass Spectrometry an Introduction, Wiley, 2003.

8. Richard B. Cole: Electro spray Ionization Mass Spectrometry, Wiley-Interscience; 1 edition (January 15, 1997)

9. www.waters.com/WatersDivision/ContentD.asp?watersit=EGOO-66YNU9.

10. http://www.appliedbiosystems.co.kr/dataDir/pds/Solvent%20for%20LCMSMS F06220923500_Solvents%20for%20LCMS.doc.

11. Comprehensive Pharmacy Review, Lippincott Williams & Wilkins; 5th edition.

12. K. Ramu, G. N. Lam, and B. Chien, Development of a High-Performance Liquid Chromatographic-Tandem Mass Spectrometric Method for the Determination of Pharmacokinetics of Co 102862 in Mouse, Rat, Monkey, and Dog Plasma, J. Chromatogr. B 2000; 749: 1-15.

13. http://www.cem.msu.edu/~reusch/VirtualText/Spectrpy/nmr/nmr1.htm

14. http://web.chem.queensu.ca/FACILITIES/NMR/nmr/chem805/PPT/NMR-H.ppt#257,1,NMR Nuclear Magnetic Resonance

15. Raymond P.W. Scott: Chromatographic Detectors, CRC; 1 edition (July 17, 1996)

16. Raymond P.W. Scott: Liquid Chromatography Column Theory, CRC; 1 edition (January 17, 1994)

17. www.ionsource.com/tutorial/chromatography/rphplc.htm#Solvents

18. http://www.mac-mod.com/pb/ace-ra-pb.html

19. http://www.waters.com/WatersDivision/pdfs/WA20769.pdf

20. FDA guidelines on Bioavailability and Bioequivalence Studies for Orally Administered Drug Products - General Considerations (21 CFR part 320).

21. Brazzell RK, Vane FM, Ehmann CW, Colburn WA. Pharmacokinetics of isotretinoin during repetitive dosing to patients. Eur J Clin Pharmacol. 1983; 24(5):695-702.

22. Colburn WA, Vane FM, Shorter HJ. Pharmacokinetics of isotretinoin and its major blood metabolite following a single oral dose to man. Eur J Clin Pharmacol. 1983; 24(5):689-94.

23. Brazzell RK, Colburn WA. Pharmacokinetics of the retinoids isotretinoin and etretinate. A comparative review. J Am Acad Dermatol. 1982 Apr; 6(4 Pt 2 Suppl):643-51.

24. Khoo KC, Reik D, Colburn WA. Pharmacokinetics of isotretinoin following a single oral dose. J Clin Pharmacol. 1982 Aug-Sep; 22(8-9):395-402.

25. Colburn WA, Gibson DM. Isotretinoin kinetics after 80 to 320 mg oral doses. Clin Pharmacol Ther. 1985 Apr; 37(4):411-4.

26. Lucek RW, Colburn WA. Clinical pharmacokinetics of the retinoids. Clin Pharmacokinet. 1985 Jan-Feb; 10(1):38-62. Review.

27. Nulman I, Berkovitch M, Klein J, Pastuszak A, Lester RS, Shear N, Koren G. Steady-state pharmacokinetics of isotretinoin and its 4-oxo metabolite: implications for fetal safety. J Clin Pharmacol. 1998 Oct; 38(10):926-30.

28. Cotler S, Chen S, Macasieb T, Colburn WA. Effect of route of administration and biliary excretion on the pharmacokinetics of isotretinoin in the dog. Drug Metab Dispos. 1984 Mar-Apr; 12(2):143-7.

29. Colburn WA, Vane FM, Bugge CJ, Carter DE, Bressler R, Ehmann CW. Pharmacokinetics of 14C-isotretinoin in healthy volunteers and volunteers with biliary T-tube drainage. Drug Metab Dispos. 1985 May-Jun; 13(3):327-32.

30. Lin HS, Barua AB, Olson JA, Low KS, Chan SY, Shoon ML, Ho PC. Pharmacokinetic study of all-trans-retinoyl-beta-D-glucuronide in Sprague-Dawley rats after single and multiple intravenous administration(s). J Pharm Sci. 2001 Dec; 90(12):2023-31.

31. Wyss R, Bucheli F. Quantitative analysis of retinoids in biological fluids by high-performance liquid chromatography using column switching. I. Determination of isotretinoin and tretinoin and their 4-oxo metabolites in plasma. J Chromatogr. 1988 Feb 26;424 (2):303-14.

32. Guiso G, Rambaldi A, Dimitrova B, Biondi A, Caccia S. Determination of orally administered all-trans-retinoic acid in human plasma by high-performance liquid chromatography. J Chromatogr B Biomed Appl. 1994 Jun 3;656(1):239-44.

33. Yokoyama H, Matsumoto M, Shiraishi H, Ishii H. Simultaneous quantification of various retinoids by high performance liquid chromatography: its relevance to alcohol research. Alcohol Clin Exp Res. 2000 Apr;24(4 Suppl):26S-29S.

34. Tzimas G, Burgin H, Collins MD, Hummler H, Nau H. The high sensitivity of the rabbit to the teratogenic effects of 13-cis-retinoic acid (isotretinoin) is a consequence of prolonged exposure of the embryo to 13-cis-retinoic acid and 13-cis-4-oxo-retinoic acid, and not of isomerization to all-trans-retinoic acid. Arch Toxicol. 1994;68(2):119-28.

35. Horst RL, Reinhardt TA, Goff JP, Nonnecke BJ, Gambhir VK, Fiorella PD, Napoli JL., Identification of 9-cis,13-cis-retinoic acid as a major circulating retinoid in plasma. Biochemistry. 1995 Jan 31;34(4):1203-9.

Chapter 5

Clinical Study to Evaluate the Efficacy and Acceptability of Antidiabetic Formulation in Patients with Non-insulin Dependent Diabetes Mellitus

C.S. Deshpande
S. Shah
R.N. Sahoo

INTRODUCTION

The appropriate long term management of hyperglycemia is critical for maintaining a normal quality of life for the person with diabetes and for preventing the individual from developing the acute and chronic complications of the disease. Reducing hyperglycemia to normoglycemic levels minimizes or prevents the microvascular and neuropathic complications but has only marginal effects on the macrovascular disease as hyperglycemia is only one of the factors responsible for the development of the latter. Therapy with lifestyle modification and a single oral antihyperglycemic agent is inadequate as it infrequently achieves target glycemic goals, and, if it does, the effect is usually not sustained.[1]

Combination of drugs with different mechanisms of action is a more rational approach to the treatment of patients with diabetes. Initial therapy might be with submaximal doses of two drugs. As the diabetic abnormalities progress, maximal concentrations of the drugs and addition of other classes of oral agents or insulin may be needed to maintain the target glycemic control.[1] But oral antihyperglycemic agents cause side effects such as weight gain, edema, gastrointestinal effects, lactic acidosis and liver toxicity and, therefore, they have to be used judiciously and are even contraindicated in certain situations.[1]

This lacuna stimulated research on plants suggested in the ayurvedic literature for the treatment of diabetes mellitus. The outcome of this research has been the elucidation of the mode of action for most of these plants. Thus, the present study was undertaken with the aim to evaluate the efficacy of the herbal formulation in lowering fasting and postprandial blood glucose levels, reducing glycosylated hemoglobin and improving the lipid profile in patients with NIDDM. The herbal preparation contains some selected herbs established for their antidiabetic potential like *Cyamopsis tetragonoloba* (guar gum),[2] *Trigonella foenum graceum* (methi),[3] *Momordica charantia*,[4] *Gymnema sylvestre*,[5] *Eugenia jambolana*,[6] *Pterocarpus marsupium*[7]. Thus, each of these plants seems to possess a different mechanism of action. Combining all these plants would result in a product that would probably help achieve glycemic control.

MATERIAL AND METHODS

Patients Selection

Twelve patients with NIDDM and the following criterion were enrolled in the study:

- fasting blood sugar ≥ 126 mg/dl but not ≥ 250 mg/dl
- glycosylated hemoglobin between 6.8 – 10%

These patients were either freshly diagnosed for NIDDM, maintained on a standard diabetic diet (at least 50% carbohydrates) or had uncontrolled NIDDM with the dose of sulphonylurea and/or biguanides not exceeding 50% of the maximum recommended dose.

The patients were of either sex in the age group of 30–70 years and with a body mass index between 80–130% of their ideal weight.

Patients suffering from diabetes mellitus for more than 15 years were not included in the trial. Similarly, patients with poorly controlled diabetes mellitus with severe hyperglycemia (FBS > 250), progressive weight loss, insulin dependency or end organ damage were not considered for inclusion in the trial. Patients on medication known to affect glucose metabolism such as glucocorticosteroids, diuretics and oral contraceptives were also not considered for inclusion in the trial. Patients having other major illness as indicated by medical history, physical examination, ECG, or routine laboratory tests were also excluded from the trial. Besides patients with impaired renal and liver function (serum creatinine ≥ 2 mg/dl and SGPT ≥ 2 times the normal value) were also excluded from the trial. Patients engaged in vigorous exercise or less than normally ambulatory or having a poor diet control in terms of a fluctuating calorie intake were not included. Pregnant or lactating women were also not considered for enrollment. An Independent Ethics Committee had approved the protocol. All the patients gave written informed consent before enrollment into the trial.

Study Design

The study was conducted as an open and multicentric trial, i.e. conducted at two sites. A detailed diabetic history was obtained for the patients recruited in the study and noted in the case report form. The diabetic history taking included inquiry into the onset, duration and course of the disease. The investigators also noted the dosage and duration of the antidiabetic medication on which the patient had been stabilized. Family history of diabetes, concomitant illness, details of the drugs/treatment taken for such illness, history of allergy to any medication and obstetric and menstrual history (in case of females) was also recorded. Patients also had to undergo a general, systemic and ophthalmic examination.

Efficacy evaluation parameters included fasting and postprandial blood sugar, glycosylated hemoglobin and lipid profile. These investigations were conducted at baseline and repeated at the end of the study, i.e. Week 11/13. During the interim follow up visits, i.e. Week 3/5 and 7/9 estimation of fasting and postprandial blood sugar was performed. Additionally at Week 7/9 estimation of glycosylated hemoglobin was performed.

Safety monitoring included CBC, urine routine, serum creatinine and SGPT that were performed at baseline and repeated at the end of the study, i.e. Week 11/13.

The investigators using a standard scale graded the subjective parameters such as polyuria, polyphagia, weakness and pain at baseline and also at the follow-up visits. At the end of the study the investigator assessed the overall efficacy and tolerability to the treatment. The dose of the investigational drug was 1 sachet thrice a day and had to be taken along with the usual OHAs (if appropriate). Compliance to the study medication was noted at every follow-up visit. The patients were instructed to contact the investigator at any time if they developed an exacerbation of any of the symptoms.

Table 5.1. Formulation

Each sachet contains:

Indian Name	Botanical Name	Quantity
Guargum	*Cyamopsis tetragonoloba*	2 g
Methi	*Trigonella foenum graecum*	1 g
Extracts of		
Karela	*Momordica charantia*	200 mg
Gudmar	*Gymnema sylvestre*	400 mg
Jamun	*Eugenia jambolana*	200 mg
Vijaysar	*Pterocarpus marsupium*	200 mg
Base		*q.s.*

Evaluation Parameters

1. Blood sugar (fasting and postprandial)
2. Glycosylated hemoglobin
3. Lipid profile
4. **Polyuria:** It was graded on a five point scale as (0 = no polyuria; 1 = 1–4 frequency in day time, 0–2 frequency in night and normal volume; 2 = 5–7 frequency in day time, 3–5 in night time with excessive volume; 3 = 8–10 frequency in day time and 6–8 frequency in night time with excessive volume; 4 = increased frequency of urination and thirst (once in 2 hours) and intake is in excessive amounts).
5. **Polyphagia:** It was graded on a five point scale as (0 = no polyphagia; 1 = two main meals + 1 light breakfast (normal quality); 2 = two main meals, and 2–3 light snacks with increased quantity; 3 = two main meals, and 2–3 light snacks (normal quality); 4 = two main meals and 3–5 light snacks with increased quantity; 5 = two main meals and more than 5 snacks with increased quantity).
6. **Weakness:** It was graded on a four point scale as (0 = routine activity without feeling of weakness; 1 = patient feels weakness during routine activity; 2 = routine activity of the patient disturbed but the patient is not bedridden; 3 = patient is hospitalized/bedridden).

7. **Pain:** It was graded on a four point scale as (0 = no pain in routine activity; 1 = pain which does not disturb routine activity; 2 = pain with slight limitations of movements disturbing the routine activity; 3 = pain with severe limitation of movements and activity reduced remarkably).

8. **Overall efficacy:** At the end of the study the overall efficacy to the treatment was assessed independently by the investigator and patient on a five-point scale (1 = excellent, i.e. when there is complete relief of symptoms; 2 = good, i.e. when there is partial relief of symptoms; 3 = fair, i.e. when there is minimal relief of symptoms; 4 = poor, i.e. when there is no relief of symptoms; 5 = very poor, i.e. when there is worsening of symptoms).

Safety Parameters

1. CBC
2. Urine routine
3. Serum creatinine
4. SGPT
5. Investigators assessment of overall tolerability: The investigator graded the overall tolerability to the investigational drug on interrogating the patient as (1 = excellent i.e. no side effects, 2 = good, i.e. mild side effects, 3 = fair, i.e. moderate side effects, 4 = poor, i.e. severe side effects requiring withdrawal from therapy).

Statistical Methods

All variables were subjected to paired t test. The null hypothesis tested was that there was no statistically significant difference among treatment groups for baseline assessments and Week 3/5, Week 7/9 and Week 11/13 assessments. All comparisons were tested at a significance level of p = 0.05.

OBSERVATIONS

Demographics and patient characteristics: Amongst the twelve patients enrolled in the study nine patients (6 males and 3 females) completed the trial while the remaining three lost to follow-up. The mean age of the nine patients who completed the trial was 44.38 ± 9.62 years. The mean weight and height of these patients were 74.56 ± 9.84 kg and 165.28 ± 9.48 cm respectively. Two of the patients were freshly diagnosed for diabetes and in the others the duration of the disease ranged from 3 months to eleven years.

Clinical efficacy results: The clinical responses of the patients were determined and the results are as shown in Tables 5.2 to 5.5.

Fasting blood sugar: The fasting blood sugar values reduced by 20.04% in 7/9 patients (77%) at Week 3/5, by 20.37% in 8/9 patients (88%) at Week 7/9 and by 25.03% in 7/8 patients (88%) at Week 11/13. The mean value for fasting blood sugar at Week 3/5 (143.44 ± 19.38), Week 7/9 (137.49 ± 18.18) and Week 11/13 (136.94 ± 34.31) were significantly different from the mean baseline value (170.72 ± 33.77) (p < 0.05).

Postprandial blood sugar: The postprandial blood sugar values reduced by 25.82% in 8/9 patients (88%) at Week 3/5, by 28.27% in 8/9 patients (88%) at Week 7/9 and by 35.52% in 6/8 patients (75%) at Week 11/13. The mean value for postprandial blood sugar at Week 3/5 (178.99 ± 59.75), Week 7/9 (178.47 ± 56.13) and Week 11/13 (167.44 ± 32.81) were significantly different from the mean baseline value (245.18 ± 90.75) (p < 0.05).

Glycosylated hemoglobin: The glycosylated hemoglobin values reduced by 18.24% in 6/8 patients (75%) at Week 7/9 and by 21.63% in 6/8 patients (75%) at Week 11/13. The mean value for glycosylated hemoglobin at Week 7/9 (7.15 ± 0.65) and Week 11/13 (7.06 ± 0.44) were significantly different from the mean baseline value (8.34 ± 1.17) (p < 0.05).

Table 5.2: Effect of treatment with antidiabetic granules in patients with NIDDM

Variable	Mean value at Baseline	Week 3/5	Week 7/9	Week 11/13
Fasting blood sugar	170.72 (224.9–126)	143.44 (167–113)*	137.49 (161.9–116.8)*	136.94 (208.5–93.3)*
Postprandial blood sugar	245.18 (374.1–120.9)	178.99 (264.2–106.6)*	178.47 (247.1–104.9)*	167.44 (234.3–128.6)*
Glycosylated Hb	8.34 (10–6.8)	-	7.15 (7.9–6.2)*	7.06 (7.8–6.5)*
Cholesterol	208.78 (251.9–175.3)	-	-	186.94 (244.2–133.6)
HDL	44.38 (53.6–35.4)	-	-	40.13 (50.8–28.9)
VLDL	33 (50–16)	-	-	27.43 (37–19)
LDL	128.57 (158–108)	-	-	125.29 (176–94)
Triglyceride	214.33 (557.5–79.7)	-	-	180.15 (486–94.3)
Polyuria	1.22 (2–1)	1 (1–1)	1 (1–1)	1 (1–1)
Polyphagia	1.89 (2–1)	1.67 (2–1)	1.67 (2–1)	1.5 (2–1)
Weakness	1.56 (2–1)	1.33 (2–1)	1.22 (2–1)	1.13 (2–1)
Pain	1.33 (2–1)	1.22 (2–1)	1.22 (2–1)	1.13 (2–1)
Weight	73.83 (88–60)	75 (87–60)	74.17 (88–59)	74.88 (89–60)

n = 8 Values are expressed as the mean (max-min)
* significantly different from baseline (p < 0.05)

Table 5.3: Effect of treatment with antidiabetic granules in patients with NIDDM

| Variable | Per cent difference from baseline at | | |
	Week 3/5	Week 7/9	Week 11/13
Fasting blood sugar	13.83 (41.5–13.77)	17.5 (45.2–5.41)	17.69 (48.62–8.64)
Postprandial blood sugar	22.63 (65.76–2.9)	18.32 (72.2–61.27)	25.38 (60.36–6.37)
Glycosylated Hb	-	11.68 (38–11.76)	13.85 (33–14.7)
Cholesterol	-	-	9.98 (39.9–3.03)
HDL	-	-	8.91 (24.54–10.38)
VLDL	-	-	10.41 (40–32.14)
LDL	-	-	2.68 (19.73–24.82)
Triglyceride	-	-	11.36 (40.08–29.33)

n = 8. Values are expressed as the mean (max-min)

Table 5.4: Effect of treatment with antidiabetic granules in patients with NIDDM

Variable	Mean value at	
	Baseline	*Week 11/13*
Hemoglobin	13.91 ± 1.46	13.41 ± 1.15
RBC	4.88 ± 0.25	4.57 ± 0.30
WBC	7912.50 ± 1759.41	7450.00 ± 1546.42
Platelets	299571.43 ± 66266.78	324125.00 ± 94573.38
Serum creatinine	0.94 ± 0.13	0.93 ± 0.09
SGPT	39.14 ± 13.98	32.28 ± 8.63

Values are expressed as the mean ± std. deviation

n = 8

Table 5.5: Overall efficacy and tolerability of treatment with antidiabetic granules
in patients with NIDDM

Response	Overall	Efficacy (Investigator)	Overall	Efficacy (Patient)	Overall Tolerability
Excellent	–		1		3
Good	4		2		5
Fair	2		3		–
Poor	–		1		–
V Poor	–		–		–

Values expressed are the number of patients reporting the response

SERUM LIPIDS

Cholesterol

The cholesterol levels reduced by 17.4% in 5/8 patients (63%) at Week 11/13. The mean value for cholesterol at Week 11/13 (186.94 ± 36.54) was not significantly different from the mean baseline value (208.78 ± 28.25).

HDL

The HDL levels reduced by 18.27% in 5/8 patients (63%) at Week 11/13. The mean value for HDL at Week 11/13 (40.13 ± 6.85) was not significantly different from the mean baseline value (44.38 ± 7.02).

VLDL

The VLDL levels reduced by 24.75% in 5/7 patients (71%) at Week 11/13. The mean value for VLDL at Week 11/13 (27.43 ± 7.5) was not significantly different from the mean baseline value (33 ± 12.68).

LDL

The LDL levels reduced by 10.84% in 5/7 patients (71%) at Week 11/13. The mean value for LDL at Week 11/13 (125.29 ± 29.97) was not significantly different from the mean baseline value (128.57 ± 21.34).

Triglycerides

The triglyceride levels reduced by 23.09% in 6/8 patients (75%) at Week 11/13. The mean value for triglyceride at Week 11/13 (180.15 ± 128.48) was not significantly different from the mean baseline value (214.33 ± 150.59).

Polyuria: The mean score for polyuria at Week 3/5 (1 ± 0), Week 7/9 (1 ± 0), and Week 11/13 (1 ± 0) were not significantly different from the mean baseline score (1.22 ± 0.44).

Polyphagia: The mean score for polyphagia at Week 3/5 (1.67 ± 0.5), Week 7/9 (1.37 ± 0.5), and Week 11/13 (1.5 ± 0.53) were not significantly different from the mean baseline score (1.89 ± 0.33).

Weakness: The mean score for weakness at Week 3/5 (1.33 ± 0.5), Week 7/9 (1.22 ± 0.44), and Week 11/13 (1.13 ± 0.35) were not significantly different from the mean baseline score (1.56 ± 0.53).

Pain: The mean score for pain at Week 3/5 (1.22 ± 0.44), Week 7/9 (1.22 ± 0.44), and Week 11/13 (1.13 ± 0.35) were not significantly different from the mean baseline score (1.33 ± 0.5).

Weight: The mean weight at Week 3/5 (75.00 ± 9.78), Week 7/9 (74.17 ± 10.26) and Week 11/13 (74.88 ± 10.37) were not significantly different from the mean weight at baseline (73.83 ± 10.75).

Overall efficacy: The overall efficacy to treatment with the investigational drug is as shown in Table 5.4.

Safety parameters: As shown in Table 5.3, no abnormalities in the laboratory tests were observed at Week 11/13. No statistically significant change in the pre and postvalues for hemoglobin, red blood cell count, white blood cell count, platelet count, serum creatinine, and SGPT was observed.

Overall tolerability: The drug was very well tolerated with no reported incidences of side effects (Table 5.4).

DISCUSSION

Early type 2 diabetes is clinically manifested as high postprandial blood glucose (PPG) levels, modestly elevated fasting blood glucose and glycosylated hemoglobin A1c (A1C) levels, and elevated serum triglyceride levels. In these patients the first-phase but not the second-phase insulin secretion by pancreatic beta cells is blunted. Therapeutic objective in these patients is twofold (1) improve insulin sensitivity in peripheral tissue, and (2) reduce the size of the glucose burden ("peaks") presented to peripheral tissues.[8]

Improvement in insulin sensitivity by *Momordica charantia* and prevention of carbohydrate absorption by Guargum, components of the herbal formulation, would help achieve these therapeutic objectives.

In late type 2 diabetes both the first-phase and second-phase insulin secretions are impaired as the pancreatic betacell failure progresses. Although profound elevations in fasting blood glucose levels characterize later diabetes, postprandial glucose elevations and the A1C levels are even higher than in early diabetes. Insulin secretion can no longer inhibit hepatic gluconeogenesis and the processes of glucotoxicity and lipotoxicity are at work.[8]

The therapeutic objective in these patients is threefold: (1) stimulate betacell insulin production (or replace it with exogenous insulin), (2) improve insulin sensitivity in peripheral tissue, and (3) increase insulin sensitivity in the liver.

Gymnema sylvestre has been reported to promote the secretion of insulin while improvement in insulin sensitivity has been observed with *Momordica charantia*.[11,14] Thus patients in the late stage of diabetes could also derive benefit from this herbal formulation.

The present study was conducted in patients with newly diagnosed or uncontrolled NIDDM wherein a significant reduction in the postprandial and fasting blood glucose (PPG) levels and glycosylated hemoglobin A1c (A1C) levels was observed.

Fasting blood glucose levels reduced significantly from 170.72 (224.9–126) at baseline to 143.44 (167–113) at Week 3/5, to 137.49 (161.9–116.8) at Week 7/9 and 136.94 (208.5–93.3) at Week 11/13 ($p < 0.05$).

Postprandial blood glucose levels reduced significantly from 245.18 (374.1–120.9) at baseline to 178.99 (264.2–106.6) at Week 3/5, to 178.47 (247.1–104.9) at Week 7/9 and 167.44 (234.3–128.6) at Week 11/13 ($p < 0.05$).

The A1C levels reduced significantly from 8.34(10–6.8) at baseline to 7.15 (7.9–6.2) at Week 7/9 and 7.06 (7.8–6.5) at Week 11/13 ($p < 0.05$).

As blood glucose control has been correlated to decreased rates of microvascular disease, the herbal formulation would be effective in preventing the microvascular complications of diabetes.[1] Tight glycemic control, however, has marginal effects on the complications of macrovascular disease (cardiovascular disease — coronary artery disease, peripheral vascular disease, stroke).[9] Elevated levels of low-density lipoprotein (LDL) cholesterol and serum triglycerides and decreased levels of high-density lipoprotein (HDL) cholesterol in patients with type 2 diabetes contribute to the development of CHD.[10]

Extensive research has demonstrated that interventions that lower LDL cholesterol and raise HDL cholesterol levels decrease CHD risk.[10]

In the present study, cholesterol levels reduced from 208.78 (251.9–175.3) to 186.94 (244.2–133.6), HDL levels reduced from 44.38 (53.6–35.4) to 40.13 (50.8–28.9), VLDL levels reduced from 33 (50–16) to 27.43 (37–19), LDL levels reduced from 128.57 (158–108) to 125.29 (176–94) and serum triglyceride levels reduced from 214.33 (557.5–79.7) to180.15 (486–94.3) in three months.

It may, thus, be suggested that the formulation would be effective in delaying or avoiding the macrovascular complications of the disease. As compared to microvascular complications, the complications of macrovascular disease are more severe and responsible for 70% of morbidity in diabetic patients.[11]

The formulation was well tolerated with no reported incidences of side effects. Laboratory parameters such as CBC, SGPT, and serum creatinine did not change significantly from the baseline values. Two patients did complaint of abdominal discomfort but these side effects were well tolerated and did not necessitate withdrawal of therapy. There were also no reported incidences of hypoglycemia.

CONCLUSION

Thus one may conclude from the present study that the herbal formulation offers a very safe method of obtaining glycemic control in patients with NIDDM without the associated risk of hypoglycemia. Besides glycemic control the formulation was also effective in reducing the blood lipid levels. The formulation may thus be used singly in newly diagnosed patients of NIDDM or in combination with OHA in uncontrolled patients to achieve the recommended therapeutic goals. Control in the blood and lipid levels would delay the microvascular and macrovascular complications of the disease. The formulation was safe and it could be used in elderly patients.

REFERENCES

1. Harold E. Lebovitz MD Oral therapies for diabetic hyperglycemia. Endocrinology and Metabolism Clinics 2001:30(4)

2. Srivastava A, Longia GS, Singh SP, Joshi LD.Hypoglycaemic and hypolipaemic effects of Cyamopsis tetragonoloba (guar) in normal and diabetic guinea pigs. Indian J Physiol Pharmacol. 1987 Apr-Jun;31(2): 77-83.

3. Ajabnoor MA, Tilmisany AK. Effect of Trigonella foenum graecum on blood glucose levels in normal and alloxan-diabetic mice. J Ethnopharmacol. 1988 Jan;22(1):45-9.

4. Day C, Cartwright T, Provost J, Bailey CJ. Hypoglycaemic effect of Momordica charantia extracts. Planta Med. 1990 Oct;56(5):426-9.

5. Sugihara Y, Nojima H, Matsuda H, Murakami T, Yoshikawa M, Kimura I. Antihyperglycemic effects of gymnemic acid IV, a compound derived from Gymnema sylvestre leaves in streptozotocin-diabetic mice. J Asian Nat Prod Res. 2000;2(4):321-7.

6. Sharma SB, Nasir A, Prabhu KM, Murthy PS, Dev G. Hypoglycaemic and hypolipidemic effect of ethanolic extract of seeds of Eugenia jambolana in alloxan-induced diabetic rabbits. J Ethnopharmacol. 2003 Apr;85 (2-3):201-6.

7. Grover JK, Vats V, Yadav S. Effect of feeding aqueous extract of Pterocarpus marsupium on glycogen content of tissues and the key enzymes of carbohydrate metabolism. Mol Cell Biochem. 2002 Dec;241 (1-2):53-9.

8. Brunton S, Lorber D, White RD. Type 2 diabetes mellitus: a practical approach to management. Greenwich CT: Monograph by the New York Medical College and QD Healthcare Group. 2001.

9. American Diabetes Association. Implications of the diabetes control and complications trial. Diabetes Care 2002;25(Suppl 1):S25-7.

10. Stratton IM, Adler AI, Neil HA, et al. Association of glycemia with macrovascular and microvascular complications of type 2 diabetes (UKPDS 35): prospective observational study. BMJ 2000;321:405-12.

11. Laakso M. Hyperglycemia and cardiovascular disease in type 2 diabetes. Diabetes 1999;48:937-42.

12. Kannel WB, McGee DL. Diabetes and cardiovascular disease: the Framingham Study. JAMA 1979;241: 2035-8.

Chapter 6

An Overview of Data Management

K.N. Bopanna

INTRODUCTION TO DATA MANAGEMENT

Clinical data management is a process that manages clinical data to produce a high quality, clean and analyzable database.

Clinical data management is a key business process in drug discovery lifecycle and our lean DM structure ensures drastic reduction in time from development to market for all phases of clinical research.

Clinical data management is the process of collecting, entering, cleaning, and reporting on data recorded in clinical trials.

Data management is involved[1-3] in all aspects of processing clinical trial data, working with a range of computer applications and database systems to support collection, cleaning and management of subject or patient data. Typically this includes:

- Input into the design of protocols, which define what data are to be collected and at what times
- Design and approval of Case Report Forms, on which subjects' data are collected
- Database design for the study, ensuring it meets requirements for data entry and reporting

Objectives

- The collected data is complete and accurate so that the results are correct.
- The trial database is complete and accurate, and a true representation of what took place in the trial.
- The trial database is sufficiently clean to support the statistical analysis, and its subsequent presentation and interpretation of the trial report.

Importance of Clinical Data Management (CDM)

- To provide consistent, accurate and valid clinical data
- To support the accuracy of the final conclusion and report
- CDM is a vital vehicle in clinical trials to ensure the integrity and quality of data being transferred from trial subjects to a database system (Fig. 6.1)

Good Clinical Data Management Practices (GCDMP)

Provide guidance on accepted practices for many areas of CDM that are not covered by existing regulations and guidance documents.
Serve multiple audiences

- Data managers, Statisticians, Site Personnel, Clinical Professionals, Compliance Auditors, Regulatory Affairs Personnel and Clinical Research Professionals

Elements of Data Management

- Data Management Plan
- CRF Processing/Filing
- Data Entry
- Validation (Query Generation and Management)
- SAE Reconciliation
- Coding
- Quality Checks
- Data Transfer

Process involved in Data Management

- Study Initiation
- Study Conduct
- Study Closure

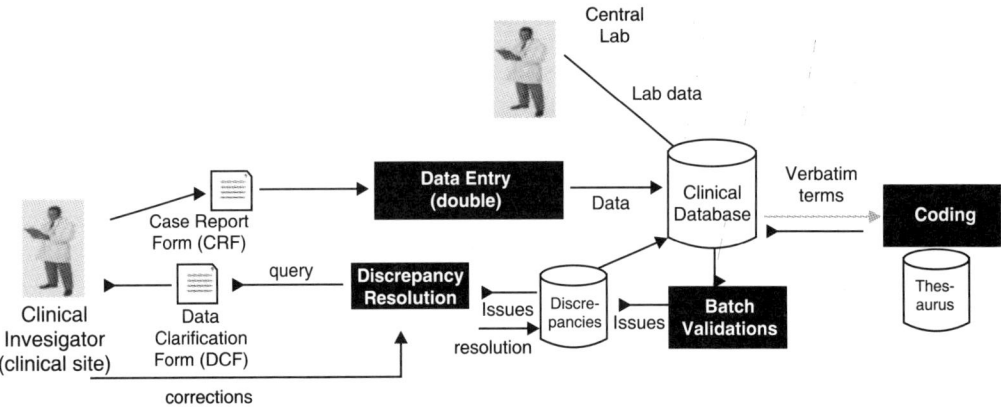

Fig. 6.1 Data flow

STUDY INITIATION

1. CRF Designing

Case Report Form (CRF) can be defined as a printed, optical or electronic document or an instrument used by the investigator/site to record all of the protocol required information to be reported to the sponsor on each trial subject, i.e. collect the relevant patient data which is used for the analysis of the investigational drug.

- Consideration should be given to what data should be collected and how the data will be used to meet the objectives of the study.
- Questions and prompts should be made specific and clear enough to assure that complete and comparable data are obtained
- Designing of CRF should be done with the primary safety and efficacy endpoints in mind as the main goal of data collection along with secondary objectives (if any).

The CRF design team is formed by the Project Manager which usually consists of Project Manager, Database Designer, Biostatistician, CRF Designer, and Clinical Trial Manager.

- Once the propobal is accepted and the contract is signed, CRF designer designs the CRF pages as per the protocol.
- The various drafts of the CRF are reviewed by the Project Manager and the biostatistician who make sure that the primary and secondary endpoints are captured in the CRF and are later sent for approval by the Sponsor.
- A Clinical Trial Manager with his vast experience gives suggestions and feedback on how the CRF should be designed.

2. CRF Annotation

CRF Annotation involves identifying the objects which are required to be created in the database to capture the data from the CRF for the study. An annotated CRF is a CRF in which the variable names are written next to the spaces provided for an investigator. It serves as a link between database and the questions on the CRF.

- Once the approval is obtained from the Sponsor, the database designer designs the database.
- Sponsor specifications for the Database/Study design, e.g. Variable Names, Codelists Names, Codelist Values, etc. should be obtained if any).
- The final version of Protocol and CRF should be used to annotate CRF.

There are different ways to annotate CRFs:

- Variable names are handwritten on a printed CRF.
- Electronically annotate using appropriate softwares e.g., PDF writer. Sharing an electronic copy of an annotated CRF is more convenient than sharing a copy of a handwritten annotated CRF (Fig. 6.2).

Annotation Guidelines e.g. in oracle clinical

- DCI: Represents the individual CRF Page
- DCM: Comprises related set of question groups
- Question Group: Comprises related questions
- Question: Identifying individual data point that needs to be captured. It could be numeric or text, etc.
- DVG Name: The fixed set of options to be chosen for the questions

An example of annotated CRF is as follows:

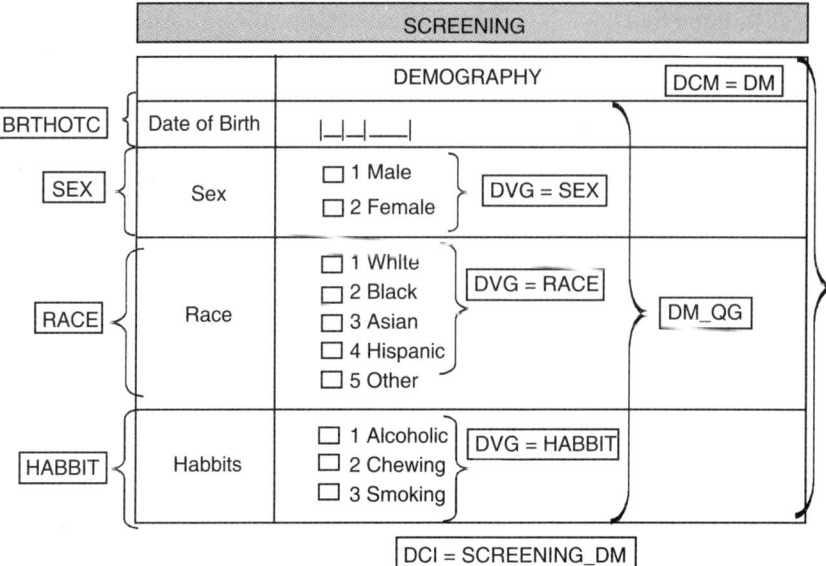

Fig. 6.2. Demographic details of participants

3. Designing Data Entry Screens

Data entry screens are designed by the database programmer for capturing the CRF data onto the database for processing the data.

- Once the annotated CRF is approved by the Sponsor, Project Manager initiates the database programming to design the data entry screens.
- Informal test is conducted on database design and data entry screens before submitting for formal validation of the same.

Validation of data entry screens

Data Entry Associate (DEA) shall validate the database using dummy patient and any issues arising during the process shall be documented and these errors shall be corrected by the database programmer subsequently. This process would continue till all the data entry screens are error-free.

4. Data Management Plan (DMP)

Clinical Data Management Plan describes the data management procedures intended to be followed for the project. These guidelines are used for processing the data to make it clean and analyzable for submission to regulatory authorities for approval.

- Data Entry/Tracking Guideline
- Data coding Guideline
- Data DCF Flow Guideline
- Data Transfer Guideline
- Non-CBF Data Handling Guideline
- Quality Control Plan Guideline
- SAE Reconciliation Guideline

- Universal Ruling Guideline
- Irresolvable Data Report Guideline

STUDY CONDUCT

1. Data Entry

This is the process of entering the CRF data onto the study database. The data entry associates carry out the entry process in an interactive blinded double entry method to ensure error-free entry.

The process involved is:

- First Pass Data Entry in which the initial keying is performed.
- Second Pass Data Entry is performed, where a second user keys the same data to ensure the accuracy and any differences should be resolved.
- Double entry has been proven to provide a 98% accuracy rate when entering data from the CRF into the database.
- Independent data entry with third party reconciliation is also an option, especially for Japanese submission.
- The first DEA (Data Entry Associate) shall key the data followed by a second, independent DEA (Data Entry Associate). The DEGL (Data Entry Group Leader) or designate shall compare the two electronic copies of data resulting from the independent data entry by reviewing a report of discrepancies.
- In the event that a discrepancy is identified, the DEGL (Data Entry Group Leader) or designate shall compare the entries to the SDD (Study Data Document) and make a decision regarding which of the entries is accurate.

2. Discrepancy Management

After Data entry is completed, data validation will be done using both manual and programmed checks.

A discrepancy is a variance between actual and expected responses as defined in the Data Validations document. Discrepancies may result from transcription errors during data entry, validation conditions arising from validation procedures, or unexpected but real clinical results.

There are four types of discrepancies (in oracle clinical):

- Univariate: Generated when data is different from that defined for the DCM questions.
- Manual and Manual Header: Generated by the operator during data entry or edit of field. Used when operator wants data validation team to look at the data. Manual discrepancies can be created during data entry (operator comment) or during discrepancy review. Manual header discrepancies can only be created during discrepancy review.
- Multivariate: Generated when data in one or more fields does not meet criteria for a validation procedure and is evaluated by the validation team.
- Indicator Discrepancy: The response to an indicator question determines which set of the remaining questions require responses.

Managing discrepancies includes identifying them, investigating their cause; resolving them or declaring them irresolvable.

If any discrepancy is identified, it is managed by the Clinical Data Coordinator (CDC) on consultation with the investigator using an instrument called Data Clarification Form (DCF).

3. SAE Reconciliation

Adverse events are classified as serious or non-serious. A serious adverse event is any AE that meets the ICH GCP definition of being:

- Fatal
- Life-threatening
- Requires or prolongs hospital stay
- Results in persistent or significant disability or incapacity
- A congenital anomaly or birth defect
- An important medical event as judged by the investigator

Serious Adverse Event (SAE) data reconciliation is to make sure that the SAE data received at Data Management is matching with the SAE data received at pharmacovigilence, i.e. reconciliation is performed to ensure that events residing in SAE database and those residing in the clinical database are consistent. It is an iterative process that occurs several times during the study. When to reconcile, is determined by the frequency of data receipt, the scheduling of safety updates, and the timing of interim and final reports.

4. Data Coding

Adverse events and medication terms in the clinical trials are crucial in analysis. Statisticians, Medical Writers, Clinical Scientists, and Medical Monitors use this data to make conclusions about the safety, and the efficacy, of investigational drugs.

The coding of medical terms is performed to maintain consistency which is used for analysis of the data. There are a number of drugs that contain the same ingredients. For easy recognition, reporting and analysis coding is done. It involves matching different medication terms containing the same entity to a specific scientific medication term of a standard dictionary. Basis for coding adverse events is similar to coding of medications. Investigators may use different names to refer to the same disease. All different terms referring to the same disease are coded to a scientific term of a standard dictionary which is recognized worldwide.

Dictionaries accepted by the pharmaceutical companies are for adverse events: MedDRA, WHO-ART, ICD, COSTART. For medications: WHO-DD, MedDRA, ICD.

STUDY CLOSURE

1. Quality Control

The purpose of this procedure is to ensure that quality is built into the clinical database for all the projects. Any difference between the data in the CRF and the database without a supporting documentation is considered an error. PDM, Biostatistician and Sponsor would be involved in finalizing the procedure of QC.

The Quality Control (QC) procedures to be followed are:

Critical QC: The purpose of the review of critical data is to ensure that a defined number of data fields, considered by sponsor and biostatistician to be crucial in determining the outcome of the study that are 100% error-free. The number of unique critical data may not exceed 20 fields.

CDC or designate will perform a 100% review of the critical data captured in database with Study Data Document (includes CRFs, Protocol Waivers (if any), DCFs). CDC shall document the results of the critical data items review on the QC Form. All errors identified will be corrected in the database.

Final QC: The purpose of the final inspection is to provide an estimate of the error rate between the SDD and the database. The final inspection is also to ensure the entire data management process, including data entry and database updates have produced a high quality database.

The PM shall use the following formula to determine the sample size:

$\sqrt{n+1}$ where n = the number of randomized subjects in the study, and the sample size does not exceed 20 subjects or 20% of the total number of subjects enrolled, whichever number is smaller.

2. Finalisation of Data Handling Report (DHR)

The document captures details on of data during the conduct of the study which differs from the process explained in the DMP.

DHR is brought to biostatistician and sponsor notice to be considered for analysis and medical writing.

Procedure

1. Create DHR
   DHR is a document that is provided to the biostatistician and sponsor prior to database closure as a part of the data management process.
2. DHR Content
   - Outstanding data issues e.g., data clarification forms or missing pages
   - Any update of coding dictionaries during the study i.e., not mentioned in the data coding guidelines
   - Any deviations from the DMP
   - Any deviations from the SOPs
   - Medical terminologies which could not be coded using medical dictionaries
   - Any other relevant or critical information
3. Finalize the IDR
   Prior to database lock, the PM shall review and authorize the final DHR. The PM shall provide the copies of the DHR to biostatistician and sponsor for review. Biostatistician shall identify any data handling issues that need to be resolved for analysis and submit these to the PM for resolution prior to database lock.
4. Filing of DHR

3. Database Lock

- Database locking is one of the last steps in the data validation.
- CDM team is responsible for the validity and completeness of the database. All the data from the investigational site received till last patient last visit of the clinical trial is validated.
- Subsequent to completion of validation, the database is prepared for locking. Locking the study database is fundamental in preventing inadvertent or unauthorized changes at the end of the study, once the final analysis and reporting of the data have begun.
- Database lock is performed once the patient data is in and deemed clean.

The different types of database lock are soft lock and freezing of the study database:

Soft lock: The purpose of soft locking a database is to prevent changes to all or a portion of the database during the conduct of the study.

Freezing the database: Freezing is performed when the data is validated. It is the highest protected data status applied to a database when all data have reached a point of no further modification.

4. Transfer of Data

Statistical Analysis System (SAS) and American Standard Code for Information Interchange (ASCII) are the format in which the data listings are submitted for regulatory approval.

The following are the team involved in finalizing the process:

- Project Manager (PM): Authorizes data transfer guidelines.
- Database Programmer: Creates the study specific data transfer guidelines, creates transfer procedures.
- Lead Biostatistician/Biostatistician: Reviews and authorizes the data transfer guidelines considering how the analysis of the data is performed.
- Sponsor: Reviews and authorizes the data transfer guidelines.

CDM Key milestones

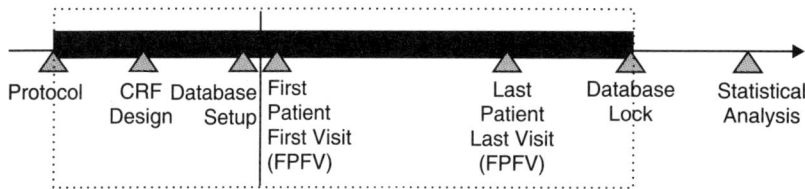

Abbreviations:

CRF	Case Report Form
DCI	Data Collection Instrument
DCM	Data Collection Module
DVG	Discrete Value Groups
DEA	Data Entry Associate
CDM	Clinical Data Management
DMP	Data Management Plan
SDD	Study Data Document
CDC	Clinical Data Coordinator
DCF	Data Clarification Form
ICH-GCP	International Conference on Harmonisation-Good Clinical Practice
PM	Project Manager
SOP	Standard Operating Procedure

REFERENCES

1. Practical guide to Clinical Data Management by Susanne Prokscha
2. Clinical Data Management by Richard K. Rondel, Sheila A. Varley, and Colin F. Webb
3. Medical Data Management by Florian Leiner, Wilhelm Gaus, Reinhold Haux, and Petra Knaup-Gregori

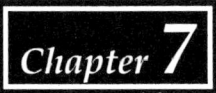

Chapter 7

Challenges and Opportunities of Clinical Research

1

S.K. Gupta
Galpalli Niranjan D.
S.S. Agarwal

Clinical research industry is growing exponentially in the past few years. It has opened a large number of career opportunities to medical, pharma and all interdisciplinary fields. Global clinical trials market is worth over US$ 45 billion and India has good potential to tap the clinical research pie. India is one of the favored destinations for clinical research by MNCs. The Indian pharma market is about $8 billion today and overall Indian pharma market is growing at 8–10%. Indian pharmaceutical industry has immense opportunities in contract research activities, clinical research, new drug delivery system, drug discovery, outsourcing for IT needs, custom synthesis, manufacturing, etc.

Clinical Research: Global Scenario

The global pharmaceutical market is estimated at US$ 427 billion and Research and Development cost is estimated at US$ 60–65 billion annually. Clinical trials involve almost 70% of time and money of new drug development. Cost of conducting clinical trials for new drug is approximately between US$ 200–250 million.

Clinical research industry has grown around the world at an unparallel rate in the past few years. It has opened up new vistas of employment for a large number of people. The clinical trials market worldwide is worth over US$ 45 billion and the industry has employed an estimated 2,10,000 people in the US and over 70,000 people in the UK and they form one-third of the total R&D staff. These large numbers can be attributed to the fact that this industry offers lucrative employment opportunities.

Clinical Trials: An Indian Perspective

India is fast emerging as a favored destination for clinical trials in new products by multinational pharmaceutical companies. Two major reasons for its popularity are:

- Easy access and availability of a large, diverse and therapy-naive population with vast gene pool
- And lower cost of technical services resulting into lowest per patient trial cost.

It is well documented that the average costs of doing Phase I/II/III drug trials in US are $20/50/100 million respectively whereas in India they are 50–60% of the same and could be up to 75% faster (Table 7.1).

India also has the advantage of having a large pool of:

- Trained doctors
- Nurses, and technical personnel
- World-class medical hospitals
- Strong information technology infrastructure
- A favorable IPR environment after signing the WTO and
- Use of English as the primary business and medical language making it an attractive option for health care companies for clinical trials. (Fig. 7.1).

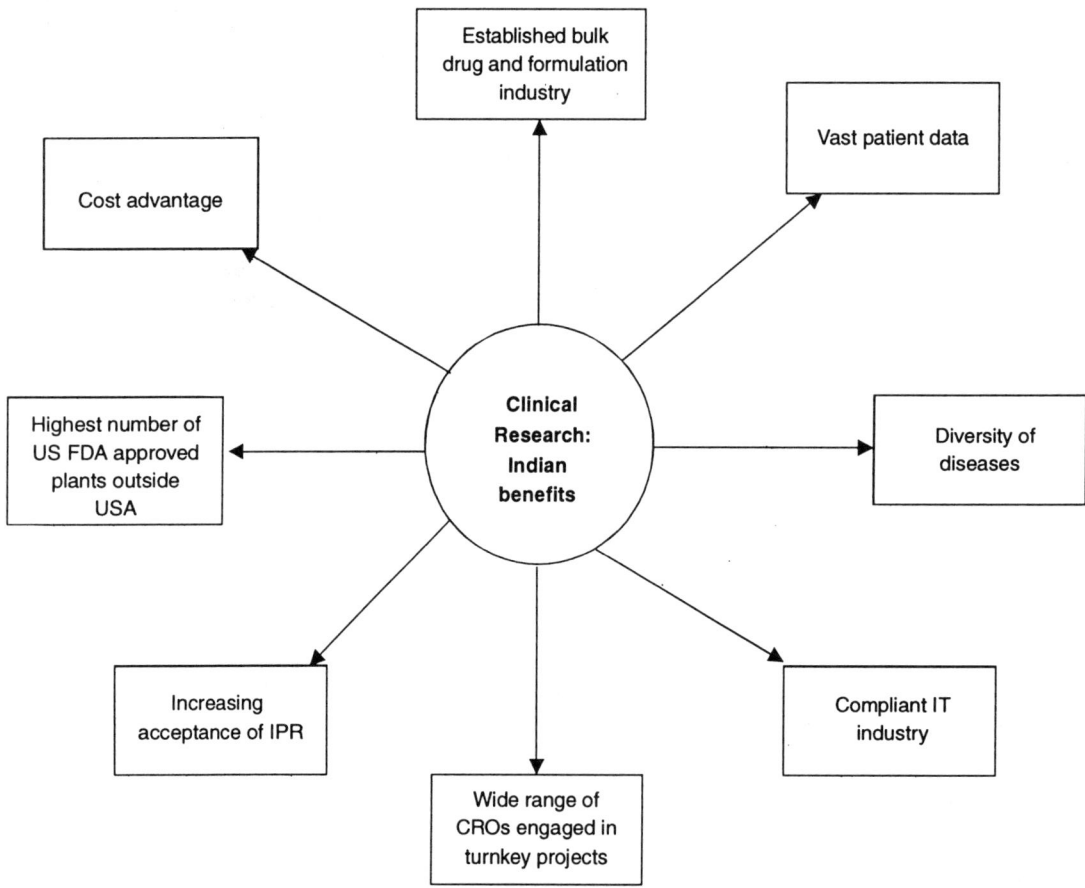

Fig. 7.1. India as an outsourcing destination

Source: Frost & Sullivan

Table 7.1: Cost of clinical trials in USA and in India

Study	Average US cost (In millions)	India cost
Phase 1	$20	50% less than the average cost in US
Phase II	$50	60% less than the average cost in US
Phase III	$100	60% less than the average cost in US

Table 7.1 shows that India can be good destination for clinical research in terms of cost and time required to conduct the clinical trials.

A number of pharmaceutical companies have successfully used clinical trial data generated from India for US FDA New Drug Application (Table 7.2).

Table 7.2: US FDA new drug application data generated from India

Company	Research molecules
Alcon	Vegamox
AstraZeneca	Merenem
Cangene	Hepatitis B Vaccine
Eli Lilly	Alimta Gemcitabine (breast cancer) Cialis (erectile dysfunction) Xygris (Septicemia)
Glaxo	Lamictal
Jannsen	Resperidal
Novartis	Tegaserod
Pfizer	Voriconazole

Source: Pharmabiz

Major Players in Clinical Research

India has numerous clinical research players with a global standard infrastructure and manpower. The number of players in the clinical research industry in India has risen to over hundred from less than eight, three years ago (Fig. 7.2).

India as a Hub for Clinical Research

1. McKinsey estimates that European and US pharmaceutical companies will spend US$1.5 billion per year on clinical trials in India by 2010.

2. Currently, there are more than 20 well-established clinical trial organizations in India with a well-developed skill set to comply with the standards such as ICH-GCP guidelines.

3. In January 2005, the government of India enacted a new rule that allows foreign pharmaceutical companies and other interested parties to conduct trials of new drugs in India at the same time that trials of the same phase are being conducted in other countries. This new rule supersedes a directive of India's Drugs and Cosmetics Rules that required a "phase lag" between India and the rest of the world.

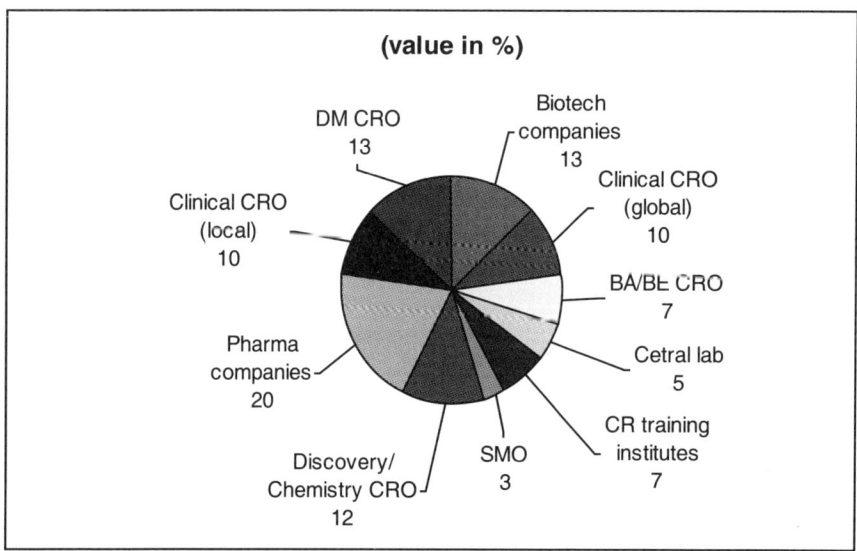

Fig. 7.2. Clinical research segmental players

4. Ranbaxy, Quintiles, Sun Pharma, Cadila, Nicholas Piramal, Lupin and many others have set up world-class clinical research centers in India to bring the drug from mind to market.
5. CDSCO in 2005 with the help of World Bank have started Pharmacovigilance system in India and is having six peripheral centers across the country.
6. Apart from Phase I–IV clinical trials, Indian companies also have large commercial opportunities in preclinical and "proof of concept studies".
7. At present there are more than 100 CROs operating in the country.
8. In India, public research institutes provide good infrastructure for conducting clinical trials. There are super specialty hospitals with state-of-the-art facilities; more that 220 medical schools, 180 dental schools, seven lakh hospital beds, and over 40 research institutes of repute. Currently, about 80 government and privately-owned Indian hospitals are engaged in global and local clinical trials with 14,000 hospitals, five lakh doctors, seven lakh beds, 162 medical colleges and 17,000 medical graduates per year.

Clinical Research in India: The Challenges

The challenges, which India face for expansion of its clinical research market, are:

1. Non-availability of sufficient number of hospital sites and trained personnel meeting ICH-GCP norms.
2. Equipments at hospitals/sites for conducting trials not always on par with trial sites in western countries.
3. Bureaucratic hurdles for regulatory approvals for global clinical trials. Approval time in India for phase I studies which is restricted to Indian molecules, is around 90 days whereas the same in western countries is about 30 days.
4. Lack of data protection for the data generated in these trials.
5. Concerns over ethical issues in patient recruitment and conduct of trial.
6. Lack of sufficient infrastructure for central laboratory services.

As of today the key issues of CRO market are consistent high quality, credibility, reliability, offering a range of services, broad and focused therapeutic expertise, timeliness, GLOCAL approach (Global Reach Local Expertise) and expertise in developing NDDS packages.

To meet the challenges and address the key issues India will have to devise policies and ensure implementation in legislative, IPR structure and regulatory issues. India also needs to help develop CROs with adequate capacity and competency in carrying out clinical research activities in compliance with ICH/GCP guidelines.

Need for Clinical Research Institutes in India

India is emerging "as hub for global clinical research". According to Mckinsey report, the global clinical trial outsourcing opportunity in India is estimated to be around Rs 5,000 crores by 2010, and there will be requirement of approximately 50,000 clinical research professionals. Today there are more than 2,50,000 positions vacant worldwide. And salaries vary from a minimum of $ 40,000 per annum for a clinical research co-ordinator to almost $100,000 per annum for a business development manager. What this means is that clinical research is definitely the next big career, and now is the time to make it a vocation.

Institute of clinical research (India) addresses the need for qualified and trained clinical research professionals by offering various programs in clinical research at its center of excellence campuses at Delhi, Mumbai and Bangalore.

ICRI is India's first and only Clinical Research institute dedicated to promoting ethical research and high-quality clinical research education in India. The courses offered by ICRI are in collaboration with Cranfield University, UK. ICRI is the only institute in India offering courses at multiple campuses throughout the country, thus giving the courses a national character.

Courses Offered

- Postgraduate diploma in clinical research
- Two years masters programme in clinical research (MSc)
- One year postgraduate diploma in clinical research
- PhD in clinical research

CONCLUSION

As the drug development is a high-risk investment, global pharmaceutical companies under pressure from stakeholders are trying to find ways for cost containment and increase the productivity. India, with its intellectual powerhouse, patient population, world-class scientific and technical skills and discipline, is an attractive destination for global players for cost and time containment. This is the reason why MNCs are outsourcing clinical research and trials to India. With Government initiatives in full swing a favorable environment is being created not only for the conduct of outsourced clinical research but also for the growth of local pharmaceutical industry at a rapid pace. With full efforts being made on the part of Government and cooperation from Indian CRO industry to meet the challenges in this field, India is set to become the *Global hub of Clinical Research.*

Importance of Clinical Research

$\boxed{2}$

Gautam Palit
Shawon Lahiri

Abstract: Peptic Ulcer Disease (PUD), one of the major gastrointestinal disorders, continues to occupy the key position in concern of both clinicians and researchers. As a result more and more drugs, both herbal and synthetic, are coming up offering newer and better options for the treatment of peptic ulcer. At the same time, each of these drugs confers simple to severe side effects, interactions and relapses. Therefore, effective anti-ulcer therapy is still lacking for which proper clinical research in evaluating the treatment schedules is necessary.

The development of a new drug from conceptual to marketing stage warrants a major commitment in both time and resources and depends upon the expertise of a wide variety of scientific, technical, clinician and managerial groups. Drug discovery and development process includes target identification, preclinical evaluation, clinical trials and postmarketing surveillance. Excellent coordination between different disciplines such as Molecular and Cellular biology, Medicinal chemistry, Pharmacology, Pharmacokinetics and Drug metabolism, development is required at each stage of this long process.

The present chapter deals with various preclinical and clinical strategies followed by evaluation of anti-ulcer drugs. From a clinical point of view, most of the anti-ulcer drugs fail at this stage due to their lack of consistency in producing long term protective effects. Therefore, the various levels at which cumulative efforts of researchers, clinicians and manufacturers are to be put, have been discussed here.

Gastrointestinal (GI) disorders affecting around a third of the world's population, are among the most common medical disorders. They encompass a spectrum of diseases and functional disturbances of the GI tract, which can vary in severity from mild and often to severe and occasionally life-threatening complications. Of these peptic ulcer is the most prevalent gastrointestinal disorder and has been a major health problem with a high rate of global incidence occurring across all ages, races and ethnicity. With pluricausal etiology which are not fully understood make peptic ulcer an important target that continues to arrest the attention of both clinicians and researchers. Peptic ulcer is believed to develop when there is a disbalance of aggressive and defensive factors either because of increased secretion of acid or pepsin or because of impairment of mucosal resistance. It involves the disruption of the mucosal integrity leading to a local defect or excavation due to active inflammation and is chronic in nature. Despite significant progress in the development of efficacious acid suppressives over the past 25 years, from histamine H2-receptor antagonists to proton pump inhibitors, this area is still of major importance. Thus, the effective and economic control of the gastric acid secretion in peptic ulcer disease that afflicts a great number of the population is still a target for drug development, refinement and pharmacological modification. Moreover, changes in gastric function can affect the bioavailability of some medications, a factor that should be borne in mind by the clinical pharmacologist when designing pharmacodynamic and pharmacokinetic protocols in the therapy of peptic ulcer disease.

Keywords: Clinical research, Peptic ulcer disease, Clinical trial

*For correspondence: gpalit@rediffmail.com

The majority of established as well as potential anti-ulcer drugs have as their therapeutic target the blockade or neutralization of gastric acid. Proton pump inhibitors (PPIs) are the most effective therapy to suppress gastric acid suppression. These agents decrease acid secretion by inhibiting parietal cell proton pumps. PPIs are substituted benzimidazole compound that is taken up by the parietal cell and converted to a sulfonamide metabolite that binds to the H^+, K^+-adenosine triphosphatase (gastric proton pump), thereby blocking all direct and indirect stimuli to acid secretion. The agents which belong to this class of drugs include omeprazole, lansoprazole, pantoprazole, esomeprazole and rabeprazole. Whereas all the PPIs currently on the market have been shown to be clinically useful, they do not all have the same pharmacological properties. Knowledge of the differences that exist in pharmacology and clinical safety and efficacy may add to the optimal use of these agents for the management of acid-related disorders. In contrast, histamine 2-receptor antagonists (H2RAs) such as ranitidine, famotidine, cimetidine, and roxatidine interfere with the histamine receptors of the parietal cell and can have their acid-inhibitory effects overcome by histamine stimulation or cholinergic drive. Whereas H2RAs reduce total 24-hour acid secretion by approximately 70%,[1] lansoprazole and other substituted benzimidazoles can achieve greater than 90% acid suppression.[2] An apparent correlation between the degree of acid inhibition by antisecretory medication and the healing of gastric ulcers suggests that the PPIs might be superior to H2RAs for gastric ulcer (GU) healing. The relative effectiveness of the PPIs compared with that of H2RAs in the treatment of patients with GUs has been examined in several clinical trials. The role of gastric mucosal cytoprotective drugs and antisecretory agents in the treatment of NSAID related gastroduodenal ulcers is less well defined. Results show that omeprazole is significantly more effective than sucralfate in inducing the healing of gastric ulcers.

Helicobacter pylori infection of the stomach has a significant clinical outcome in about 30% of affected individuals, resulting in peptic ulcer, gastric cancer and in some rare cases, lymphoma.[3] Triple and quadruple therapies have become the standard for *H. pylori* eradication. First-line treatment now consists of triple therapies with a PPI and two antibiotics out of clarithromycine, amoxicilline and metronidazole. The twice-daily dosing schedule is relatively simple and side effects are generally mild. The main alternative to PPI triple therapy is quadruple therapy, consisting of classical bismuth triple therapy (bismuth, metronidazole and tetracycline) plus a PPI. In many countries, this is now the treatment of choice for treatment failures. It leads to high eradication rates when given for seven days and can overcome metronidazole resistance[4, 5]. A capsule containing bismuth, metronidazole and tetracycline is under clinical study[4, 6]. This combination drug allows significant simplification of the dosing schedule for quadruple therapy and is likely to expand the use of this treatment. But there are difficulties with compliance of patients with the established regimens and an identifiable increase in antibacterial resistance. Hence, the problems caused by this infection are still very much with us and research and development will have to meet the challenge of evaluating new therapies or drug combinations, as well as vaccines. Another factor of importance to clinical pharmacologists is that the local inflammation produced by this organism in the stomach can potentially alter drug absorption of a number of therapeutic agents in the gastric compartment.

There are always associated risks in prescribing any drug, and this is exemplified by the commonly used non-steroidal anti-inflammatory drugs (NSAIDs). A significant number of patients on NSAIDs will develop serious complications involving the gastrointestinal tract leading to erosion and bleeding[7, 8]. Assessment of these side effects is important, not least in the development of the newer class of agents in this arena, the COX-2 selective inhibitors or *coxibs*[9–11]. Indeed, the platform for the clinical and commercial success of these latter agents has been built on the premise that they are far less injurious to the gut. But recently it was observed that COX-2 inhibition produces significant cardiac complications thus leading to the ban of selective COX-2 inhibitors. Therefore, newer agents to challenge the supremacy of these claims include the nitric oxide (NO)-donating NO-NSAIDs, also known as CINODs (cyclo-oxygenase inhibiting nitric oxide donating agents), and the dual cyclo-oxygenase-lipoxygenase inhibitors, all of which are undergoing ever-rigorous evaluation for effects on both the stomach and small intestine.

Thus, evaluation of the side effect profile of a range of new chemical entities on the gastrointestinal tract has become an issue of ever-increasing importance and more rigorous assessment in appropriately designed studies is becoming a necessity for several new classes of drug. Moreover, peptic ulcer disease is a chronic relapsing disease. There is no drug marketed that has convincingly been found to alter the natural course of this disease. Ulcer recurrence is inevitable and thus physicians need to administer the drug continuously after healing to maintain an ulcer-free state. So the need for competent clinical research has long been recognized in this field of study.

Preclinical Research and Development

Drug development is an extremely costly, time-consuming and difficult endeavor. Very few compounds survive preclinical tests and go on to clinical trials and only a very small fraction of these compounds become medically successful marketed drugs. During preclinical research and development, pharmacological characterization — including determinations of the mode of action, safety studies, effect on organs other than the gastrointestinal tract, pharmacokinetics and pharamcodynamics, mutagenicity, teratogenicity and toxicological profile — yields estimates for a clinical dose.

Pharmacological Characterization

The pharmacological class of the test drug must be identified and the mechanism of action must be established in order to determine the relation between the mechanism of action and the potential use of the drug for the treatment of peptic ulcer disease. For example, if a drug is a gastric secretory inhibitor, the mechanism of this inhibition, in so far as acid secretion should be well established[12, 13]. Comparative preclinical studies should be performed with reference standards to determine whether this drug should belong to well-established pharmacological classes of gastric secretory inhibitors such as anti-cholinergic, histamine receptor antagonists or proton pump inhibitors. Studies should be conducted to characterize effects of these drugs on other gastroduodenal physiological functions of the mucosa in order to understand whether the drug inhibits acid secretion by one or more mechanisms unrelated to those of well-known inhibitors of gastric acid secretion. For compounds possessing pharmacological actions other than inhibition of acid secretion the relative degree of specificity of these effects should be established like the cytoprotective agents including the prostaglandins that stimulate bicarbonate secretion and mucin secretion by the gastric mucosa and also increase gastric mucosal blood flow thus ameliorating ulcer.

In all these studies, investigations of a dose-response relationship with respect to the primary mechanism of action should be established. Pharmacokinetic and metabolic studies should also be conducted to provide an idea of the extent of absorption, distribution, metabolism and excretion in one or more species that is more relevant to humans.

Safety and Efficacy

Information should be provided regarding the test drug's safety including their metabolites, safety pharmacodynamics, efficacy and dose response. Description of the possible risks and adverse drug reactions to be anticipated on the basis of prior experiences with the product under investigation and with related products.

Pharmacokinetics and Product Metabolism

A summary of information on the pharmacokinetics of the investigational product should be presented including the following:

- Pharmacokinetics (including metabolism, absorption, plasma protein binding, distribution and elimination).
- Bioavailability of the investigational product using a reference dosage form
- Interactions, e.g.: product-product interaction and effects on food.

Toxicological Characterization

The potential toxicity and/or effects on other organ systems (cardiovascular, renal, hepatic, respiratory, etc.) should be identified during the pharmacological characterization of the drug. The dose used in the broad pharmacological studies should be sufficiently large multiple of the effective gastric anti-secretory, cytoprotective and anti-ulcer dosages. The difficulty, however, arises when the preclinical findings are not very clear or are of dubious clinical relevance. Then appropriate safety studies including mutagenicity and teratogenicity examinations are required. Because, anti-ulcer drugs are usually administered for long periods of time, long term, 2-year toxicity and carcinogenicity studies are also required for phase II/II of clinical development, but these studies are not needed for early clinical investigations which are usually short term (4–12 weeks of treatment).

Typical Core Studies Conducted during Clinical Development of an Anti-ulcer Drug

Clinical trial of drugs is a randomized single or double blind controlled study in human subjects designed to evaluate prospectively the safety and effectiveness of new drugs or formulation. The clinical research and development is carried out in sequential phases.

Phase I: The primary purpose of phase I studies is to establish the safety of the maximum tolerated dose in healthy adults of both sexes; to establish the safe dose range, pharmacological, pharmacokinetic and pharmacodynamic effects and adverse reactions, if any, with their intensity and nature in healthy subjects.

Phase II: Initial efficacy studies are performed in phase II utilizing controlled trials in a limited number of patients around 50–200 patients of both sexes to determine therapeutic uses, effective dose range and further evaluation of safety and pharmacokinetic when necessary.

Phase III: The purpose of these trials is to obtain adequate data about the efficacy and safety of drugs in a larger number of patients of both sexes in multiple centres usually in comparison with a standard drug and/or a placebo if a standard drug does not exist for the disease under study. On successful completion of phase III trials permission is granted for marketing of the drug.

Phase IV: After approval of the drug for marketing, postmarketing surveillance is undertaken to obtain additional information about the drug's risks, with reporting of adverse reactions, survey sampling, testing and inspection, benefits and optimal use.

Human studies designed to evaluate the safety, effectiveness or usefulness of an intervention includes research on therapeutics, diagnostic procedures and preventive measures. It is clearly accepted that it is essential to carry out research on human subjects to discover better medical and therapeutic modalities for the benefit of mankind. It is equally clear that such research on normal subjects and patients is associated with some degree of risk to the individual concerned. Certain guidelines have been framed to carry out the evaluation of drugs on human subjects in accordance with the basic ethical principles. Some of them are as follows:

Single Dose Acute Safety and Tolerance Study in Healthy Subjects

The initial study in phase I development will examine the safety and tolerance of the test drug by studying the effect of single escalating doses in order to achieve a dose that produces definitive adverse effects.

Multiple Tolerance Study on Healthy Subjects

Multi dose tolerance study should be conducted only when there is confirmation regarding the pharmacological aspect of the drug in relevance to peptic ulcer disease. For example, in the case of a drug that is believed to work via an inhibitory effect on gastric acid secretion, it would be useful to determine the dose levels and the intervals between doses that had varying and graded effects on acid production at various times during a single 24-hours period. It would be very useful to establish the nature of the gastric antisecretory action against different physiological stimuli of gastric acid secretion such as gastrin, histamine and cholinergic mediated secretory responses.

Absolute Bioavailability Studies

For drugs acting systemically, pharmacokinetics and characterization of the bioavailability of the dosage form should be performed. But for some drugs that seem to act locally on the gastroduodenal mucosa and thus are not absorbed except for a small amount of aluminium and bismuth in drugs such as sucralfate and bismuth salts, standard pharmacokinetic studies are obviously not relevant.

Drug Interaction Studies

It would be important to conduct initial drug interaction studies in healthy subjects to establish the degree of drug interaction and the possible adverse effects, if any, from such interaction and also to confirm the preclinical data and to provide an understanding of the type of patients to be selected in phases II and III of clinical development.

Placebo Controlled Trials

The need for clear demonstration of activity of the new drug cannot be avoided. This is best done when the drug is compared to a placebo. The placebo must be indistinguishable from the test drug and administered on the same predetermined dose schedule. The ideal study recommended by the FDA draft guideline would consist of four arms: placebo, active control drug and two levels of test drug. For practical reasons this type of trial is difficult to implement so an alternative approach taken is to split such a trial into two studies: placebo and one dose of test drug and two doses of test drug and an active control.

Dose Response Studies

Because a direct correlation between a pharmacological effect (i.e. acid suppression or cytoprotection) and drug efficacy (i.e., healing an ulcer) cannot yet be made, only through clinical efficacy trials in which varying doses of the study drug are used can a dose-response relationship for ulcer healing can be determined. It is very important to find an optimal dose which can be defined as the dose above which no additional efficacy occurs and below which efficacy is unlikely.

Number of Trials Needed to Determine Efficacy

The purpose of multiple trials is to ensure valid and reliable results to prove clinical efficacy. The exact numbers of trials depend on endpoints evaluated and the consistency of the results, although as a minimum, two well-controlled, double-blind, randomized trials are usually necessary to establish the safety and efficacy of a drug.

Patient Population

The number and diversity of the patients studied in clinical efficacy should be broad enough that adequate information can be obtained in terms of both efficacy and safety. For example, patients selected for entry should not only have evidence of an ulcer but also have associated symptoms so that determinations can be made during the trial of symptom response as well as ulcer healing.

Clinical Evaluation of Herbal Remedies and Medicinal Plants

Natural products and their derivatives have historically been invaluable as a source of therapeutic agents to treat various human diseases including PUD[14]. Roughly 50% of new chemical entities introduced during the past two decades are from natural products. It has long been recognized that natural product structures have the characteristics with high chemical diversity, biochemical specificity and other molecular properties that make them favorable for drug discovery. Most of the marketed established anti-ulcer drugs show incidence of relapses as their side effects. In order to overcome these adverse effects, investigation has been extended towards the search for new and novel molecules from natural resources aiming to have better and safer treatment strategy. Various natural products of plant origin — *Allophylus serratus*[15], *Desmodium gangeticum*[16], *Ocimum sanctum*[17], *Azadirachta indica*[18], *Hemidesmus racemosus*[19], *Asparagus racemosus*[20], etc. have been reported to possess anti-ulcer activity. Despite their success, research into natural products in the pharmaceutical industry has declined owing to issues such as lack of compatibility of traditional natural products extract libraries with high throughput screening. However, recent technological advances have helped to address these issues and efforts should be directed towards the isolation and characterization of the active principles and elucidation of the structure activity. As per the regulatory requirements, they may be put to clinical trials, after conducting preclinical pharmacological and toxicological studies, which may, in future, be tried for selective targeting or delivery.

All the general principles of clinical trials described earlier pertain also to herbal remedies and medicinal plants that are to be clinically evaluated for use. When an extract of a plant or a compound isolated from the plant has to be clinically evaluated for a therapeutic effect not originally described in the texts of traditional systems or, the method of preparation is different, it has to be treated as a new substance or new chemical entity and the same type of acute, subacute and chronic data will have to be generated as required by the authority before it is cleared for clinical evaluation. It should undergo all regulatory requirements before being evaluated clinically. Clinical trials with herbal preparations should be carried out only after these have been standardized and markers identified to ensure that the substances being evaluated are always the same.

The overall aim of clinical research is to provide a clear understanding of the possible risks and adverse reactions and of the specific tests, observations and precautions that may be needed for a clinical trial. This understanding should be based on the available physical, chemical, pharmaceutical, pharmacological, toxicological and clinical information on the investigational products. Clinical research in gastrointestinal disorders is now focused on the role of *H. pylori* and *H. pylori* eradication in the treatment of several upper gastrointestinal disturbances such as non-ulcer dyspepsia, ulceration during therapy with aspirin or other anti-inflammatory drugs, the treatment of precancerous conditions of the stomach, and the prevention of gastric cancer. Thus, clinical research advances will have an immense impact on the management of digestive diseases.

REFERENCES

1. Feldman M, Richardson CT. Total 24-hour gastric acid secretion in patients with duodenal ulcer. *Gastroenterology.*1986; 90:540–544.

2. Howden CW, Hunt RH. The relationship between suppression of acidity and gastric ulcer healing rates. *Aliment Pharmacol Ther.* 1990; 4:25–33.

3. Logan RP, Walker MM. ABC of the upper gastrointestinal tract. Epidemiology and diagnosis of *Helicobacter pylori* infection. *BMJ* 2001; 323: 920–922.

4. Laine L, Hunt R, El Zimaity HM, Nguyen B, Osato M, Spenard J: Bismuth-based quadruple therapy using a single capsule of bismuth biskalcitrate, metronidazole, and tetracycline given with omeprazole versus omeprazole, amoxicillin, and clarithromycin for eradication of *Helicobacter pylori* in duodenal ulcer - patients: a prospective, randomized multicenter, North American trial. *Am J Gastroenterol.* 2003; 98:562–567.

5. Katelaris PH, Forbes GM, Talley NJ, Crotty B: A randomized comparison of quadruple and triple therapies for *Helicobacter pylori* eradication: the Quadrate study. *Gastroenterology.* 2002; 123:1763–1769.

6. O'Morain C, Borody T, Farley A, de Boer WA, Dallaire C, Schuman R, Piotrowski J, Fallone CA, Tytgat G, Megraud F et al.: Efficacy and safety of single-triple capsules of bismuth biskalcitrate, metronidazole and tetracycline, given with omeprazole, for the eradication of *Helicobacter pylori*: an international multicentre study. *Aliment Pharmacol Ther.* 2003; 17:415–420.

7. Langman M, Weil J, Wainwright P, *et al.* Risks of bleeding peptic ulcer associated with individual non steroidal anti-inflammatory drugs. *Lancet* 1994; 343: 1075–1078.

8. Singh G, Triadafilopoulos G. Epidemiology of NSAID-induced gastrointestinal complications. *J Rheumatol* 1999; 26(Suppl 56): 18–24.

9. Silverstein FE, Faich G, Goldstein J, *et al.* Gastrointestinal toxicity with celecoxib *vs* non steroidal anti-inflammatory drugs for osteoarthritis and rheumatoid arthritis: the CLASS study: a randomized controlled trial. Celecoxib Long-term Arthritis Safety Study. *JAMA* 2000; 284: 247–1255.

10. Bombardier C, Laine L, Reicin A, *et al.* Comparison of upper gastrointestinal toxicity of rofecoxib and naproxen in patients with rheumatoid arthritis. VIGOR Study Group. *N Engl J Med* 2000; 343: 1520–1528.

11. Mamdani M, Rochon PA, Juurlink D, *et al.* Observational study of upper gastrointestinal haemorrhage in elderly patients given selective cyclo-oxygenase-2 inhibitors or conventional non-steroidal anti-inflammatory drugs. *Br Med J* 2002; 325: 624–627.

12. Dajani EZ, Perspectives on the pharmacology of misoprostol. In: Szabo S, Pfeifer C, eds. Ulcer disease: new aspects of pathogenesis and pharmacology. Boca Raton, Fla: CRC Press.1989; Chap. 27, 321–34.

13. Dajani EZ, Driskill DR,Bianchi RG, Collins PW, Pappo R. SC-29333, a potent inhibitor of canine gastric secretion. *Dig Dis Sci* 1976; 21:1049–57.

14. Koehn FE, Carter GT. The evolving role of natural products in drug discovery. *Nat Rev* 2005; 4:206–20.

15. Dharmani P, Mishra PK, Maurya R, Cahuahan VS, Palit G. *Allophylus serratus*: a plant with potential anti-ulcerogenic activity. *Jrnl Ethanopharmacol* 2005 (in press).

16. Dharmani P, Mishra PK, Maurya R, Cahuahan VS, Palit G. *Desmodium gangeticum*: a plant with potent anti-ulcerogenic effect. *Indian Jrnl Experimental Bio.*2005 (in press).

17. Dharmani P, Kumar KV, MAurya R, Sharma S, Srivastava S, Palit G. Evaluation of anti-ulcerogenic and ulcer healing properties of *Ocimum sanctum* Linn. *Jrnl Ethanopharmacol* 2004; 93:197–206.

18. Bandyopadhyay U, Biswas K, Chatterjee R, Bandopadhyay D, Chattopadhyay I, Ganguly CK, Chakraborty T, Bhattacharya K, Banerjee RK. Gastroprotective effects of Neem (*Azadirachta indica*) bark extract: Possible involvement of H+ K+ ATPase inhibition and scavenging of hydroxyl radical. *Life Sci* 2002; 71:2845–65.

19. Anoop A, Jegadeesan M. Biochemical studies on the anti-ulcerogenic potential of *Hemidesmus indicus* R.Br. var.indicus. *Jrnl Ethanopharmacol* 2003; 84:149–56.

20. Sairam K, Priyambda S, Aryya NC, Goel RK. Gastroduodenal ulcer protective activity of *Asparagus racemosus*; an experimental, biochemical and histological study. *Jrnl Ethanopharmacol* 2003; 86:1–10.

Chapter 8

Ethics in Clinical Research

| 1 |

Mita Nandy

Ethics is an integral part of pharmaceutical development. The main ethical dilemmas are related to balancing the needs and rights of the individual against those of society. Government-appointed regulators and investigational site staff, who are involved in every study we conduct in humans, have to be reviewed by an independent ethics committee. All developed countries have laws and codes which cover the composition of ethics committees, for instance, the need to include lay people, both sexes, representatives independent of the institution conducting a trial and a racial composition that reflects the local population.

HISTORICAL OVERVIEW

Ethical declarations can be traced back to the 5th Century BC and the Hippocratic Oath, which contains medicine's earliest ethical precept: "As to diseases, make a habit of two things — to help, or at least to do no harm". In addition, the Oath already mentions confidentiality/data protection issues:

The ethical principles governing modern medical experimentation in human subjects were first defined in the Nuremberg Code in 1947. The code, which was prompted by the atrocities committed by Nazi physicians and researchers during World War II, emphasizes the importance of voluntary consent, avoidance of unnecessary suffering and observance of high scientific standards.

Even after the Nuremberg Code was issued, however, unethical practices persisted. One infamous example, which occurred in the United States, is known as the Tuskegee case. Although penicillin had become widely available as an effective treatment for syphilis by the early 1950s, the men who participated in the Tuskegee (Alabama) syphilis study, which had begun in 1932, were not treated but merely observed until the details of the study became public in 1972. Widespread consternation ensued, and as a result the National Research Act of 1974 was passed by the US Congress. The Act created the National Commission for the Protection of Human Subjects of Biomedical and Behavioral Research, which published the Belmont Report in 1979. The Belmont Report identified three fundamental ethical principles: respect for persons, beneficence and justice, again reiterating the need to protect research subjects from abuses.

Well before the publication of the Belmont Report, in 1964, the World Medical Association developed the declaration of Helsinki as a statement of ethical principles to provide guidance to physicians and other participants in medical research involving human subjects. This declaration has since been updated five times, most recently in October 2000 at the 52nd World Medical Association General

Assembly in Edinburgh, Scotland, and is used worldwide as the most important reference document guiding ethics in research on human subjects.

Nowadays, ethical principles are embedded in, and repeated across, a plethora of Good Clinical Practice (GCP) regulations and guidelines. The Food and Drug Administration (FDA) in the United States took the lead in the 1970s, following the passage of the National Research Act which mandated the establishment of institutional review boards to review all federally funded human research.

In Europe, individual countries undertook the first initiatives, each of them creating its own regulations and/or guidelines for conducting research in human subjects. Then, in 1990, the European Union's Committee for Proprietary Medicinal Products (CPMP) published a guideline on Good Clinical Practice for trials on medicinal products in the European Community, which was the first unified standard covering all aspects of medical research in Europe. This guideline became a model for modern GCP guidance documents, and as a result non-EU countries, including Switzerland, have since issued similar guidelines that are aligned with EU provisions.

In the face of increasing globalization, an international effort was launched in the 1990s to harmonize GCP standards in the world's three major pharmaceutical-producing regions, North America, the European Union and Japan. These efforts resulted in the publication of a common document in 1996, the ICH (International Conference on Harmonisation) Harmonized Tripartite Guideline for Good Clinical Practice, which encompasses ethical principles that have their origin in the Declaration of Helsinki.

The Legal Force of Ethical Declarations and Related Regulations

The legal force of ethical declarations and related regulations on the conduct of clinical trials in human subjects — whether they are patients or healthy subjects — varies from country to country.

In some countries, such as France, Spain, the Netherlands and Japan, they have the full force of law. In the United States, CFR have legal force, but the FDA also issues guidance documents. These documents do not have any legal force as such, but could be enforceable by law on the grounds that they are "state-of-the-art" guidelines and infringements therefore constitute gross negligence. Yet other countries, notably the United Kingdom and the Nordic countries, have issued or ratified guidelines, which have not been incorporated into any legal framework. Finally, it should be noted that the Declaration of Helsinki, which is maintained and published by the World Medical Association, has nowhere attained the force of law, even though in the public mind it remains the most relevant guide to ethical behavior in human research.

Recent Developments

The European Union has now incorporated the ICH GCP guideline into the EU Clinical Trials Directive, which was approved in December 2000 by the European Parliament.

The ethical approval system in Europe also came under close scrutiny during the drafting of the clinical trial directive. Because each member state has evolved its own system of ethical approval, submitting a research protocol for ethical review in Europe has become a complex and time-consuming process, and harmonisation of this process has therefore been high on the agenda of European regulators, politicians and the pharmaceutical industry. The new EU directive marks a positive step towards harmonisation by requiring a single ethics committee opinion per country. Furthermore, the European Commission intends to draft detailed guidance for the further harmonisation of application formats and documentation for ethics committee submissions.

The recent adoption of important ethical legislation in the European Union, the guidance provided by the ICH and the latest amendment to the Declaration of Helsinki, in October 2000, have all coincided to move 'ethics' to the forefront of attention in the clinical trials community. This is reflected in a January 2001 editorial in the Journal Applied Clinical Trials, which states that 'ethics issues have moved from discussion to action'.

However, debate continues on many ethical issues, notably the use of placebo controls, the acceptability of conducting trials in children to develop pediatric formulations or dosage strengths and the testing of new Alzheimer's drugs in patients suffering from this disease who are not competent to give their personal informed consent, e.g. because they are mentally incapacitated. Other focal points of debate include medical research in the developing world, the use of genetic information and data protection.

The Consensus on the Use of Placebo

The Declaration of Helsinki states that new drugs should be tested against the best available treatments or active controls, based on the view that it is unethical to give a placebo to a patient when an effective treatment exists.

Some authorities, including the FDA, take an opposing view. There is a consensus in the pharmaceutical industry and among regulators that placebo-controlled clinical trials are not justified in patients suffering from life-threatening diseases or where the use of placebo could cause discomfort to patients and an approved treatment is already available. There is also a consensus that a placebo should not be used under the above conditions in children or mentally incapacitated adults, e.g. patients with Alzheimer's disease.

However, there is also agreement among researchers and regulators, notably the FDA, that the use of placebo is the method of choice when the disease under investigation is characterized by a high placebo response.

Thanks to rigorous placebo-controlled trials, a long list of established medicines have been discovered over the past 50 years to have no pharmaceutical effect. Placebo-controlled trials are assumed to be ethically and scientifically justified as long as the medical rationale does not affect patients' rights and the availability of alternative therapies is clearly communicated to patients and spelled out in the informed consent form.

Still, drug makers now forego placebo-controlled trials whenever possible, unless the regulatory authorities expressly require that such trials be performed. Given the new possibilities being opened up in clinical testing by pharmacogenetics, this trend will increase (see "The tailor-made medicine of tomorrow").

How to Protect the Vulnerable Subjects

Much attention has been devoted to strengthening the safeguards for vulnerable subjects, such as children and the mentally ill, e.g. Alzheimer's patients.

It is widely accepted that too little detailed prescribing guidance is available to pediatricians. The FDA has tried to improve this situation by providing commercial incentives (patent extensions) for pharmaceutical companies to produce such guidance. To obtain the necessary data, however, properly controlled clinical trials have to be conducted in children, and such studies inevitably raise ethical issues regarding patient recruitment and the impossibility of obtaining fully informed patient consent.

The discussion as to whether or not clinical research should be allowed in patients who are incapable of giving legally effective informed consent has been going on for a number of years. That effective new Alzheimer's drugs, for example, can be developed only if testing is permitted in the population of interest goes without saying. The current view is that such research should be allowed only if there is a direct benefit for the patients concerned. The legally authorized representatives of such patients may give their consent, but only in accordance with the patients' presumed will.

However, exactly how one should establish the presumed will of an incapacitated patient remains to be determined. Moreover, obtaining informed consent from a legally authorized representative presents a formidable practical obstacle. For unconscious, and even for mentally incapacitated patients, it is rare that a legal representative has been appointed. From a legal standpoint, then, one cannot simply assume that a patient's next of kin is empowered to consent on the patient's behalf. This raises an ethical dilemma: from a medical standpoint, it might be in a patient's best interests to include him/her in a clinical trial, thus giving the patient access to a new, potentially promising therapy, but from a legal standpoint, failure to obtain effective informed consent violates a key requirement of GCP. This issue is still a subject of passionate debate among ethicists, lawyers and physicians.

Studies in the Developing World

In the developed world, many patients insist upon receiving the best proven treatment available. In developing countries, by contrast, individuals, and governments, often do not have the money to pay for the most appropriate medicine or any form of treatment. For patients in the third world, participating in clinical trials is often the only way to gain access to promising drug treatments.

The problems confronting the sponsors of clinical trials in developing countries are by no means negligible, however, and the charge that drug makers merely offer a bit of token aid to the poorest of the poor in order to test their products as simply and cheaply as possible is completely off the mark.

Sponsors should not make any geographic distinctions in the design or ethical standards of its clinical trials, regardless of whether they are conducted in the "developing world" or western countries. The ICH GCP guideline is applied internationally in all our clinical trials, and is augmented by each country's specific legal requirements. It should be noted here that many trials are multi-centre, multi-national projects. In such cases, the same protocol and the same standards are used throughout the study and at all locations, thus ensuring uniform levels of compliance and patient protection.

In point of fact, conducting clinical trials in third world countries involves increased expenditures because of the decrepit or completely underdeveloped healthcare systems found there. The availability of hospitals and qualified medical personnel is limited in these countries, and hygienic conditions alone often make it all but impossible to provide medical care that is up to western standards.

The latest version of the Declaration of Helsinki states that "at the conclusion of [a] study the subjects should be assured of access to the best proven therapeutic methods identified by the study" until it is approved for marketing in their country.

Biotechnology Products and Genetic Information

There are no fundamental differences in the ethical issues raised by the testing of biotechnology products versus traditional chemical entities. A biotechnology product may require greater due diligence with respect to handling, but the ethical principles of patient care, avoidance of unnecessary suffering, informed consent and observance of high scientific standards (risk-benefit analyses) remain the same.

There are many ethics issues surrounding genotyping in clinical trials, including the right of the patient to receive or not to receive the results of genotyping. Another issue relates to the procedures used to maintain the confidentiality of genotyping results.

Data Protection

Data protection and patient confidentiality issues have been widely discussed in recent years. In Europe, a directive on data protection was approved in 1995 and became effective in 1998. Under the directive, personal data may only be collected and processed with the person's explicit consent and only for the purpose for which it is required. It is the conduct of each individual clinical team that forms the cornerstone of ethical clinical practice. Adequate and ongoing peer review within cross-functional teams is also a key prerequisite for maintaining high ethical standards.

The concept of the inviolability of the human person constitutes the basic tenet of biomedical ethics. Four main principles ensue: the principles of autonomy, of nonmaleficience, of beneficence and of justice. Some rules derive from them, for instance veracity, confidentiality, fidelity and respect of intimacy with regard to the subject of an experiment. From a practical standpoint, the design of a clinical trial must be scientifically sound otherwise it cannot be ethical. An informed consent must be obtained, in written form, from the subject in a clinical trial and he must be aware of his right to withdraw from it at any moment, Moreover, the clinical trial must be monitored throughout its duration with respect to ethics. An ethics of the methodology of clinical trials must therefore exist. Ethics in research should be a way of thinking and behaving, inherent to the research training. The researcher should be keenly conscious of the ethical requirements involved in his work, if he wishes to avoid eventual external interventions.

Overview of the Presentation

- What is ethics?
- Why must clinical trial be ethical?
- What is the aim of ethics?
- Moral problems in clinical research
- Guidelines applicable to research
- Ethical framework: 7 principles
- What makes clinical research ethical?
- Questions yet to be answered

What is Ethics?

Ethics... is the moral limitation placed on power.

– Al Jonsen

Morality

Social conventions [beliefs and practices] about right and wrong human conduct that are so widely shared that they form a stable community consensus.

Ethics (Table 8.1)

A systematic reflection on and analysis of morality
A generic term for various ways of understanding and examining the moral life.

What is the Moral Problem in Clinical Research?

Purpose of clinical research

- Is generation of knowledge about human health and illness and/or increase understanding of human biology.
- Benefit to participants, although it often occurs, is *not* the purpose of research
- People are the means to developing useful knowledge; and are thus at risk of exploitation

Table 8.1: Difference between ethics and law

Law	*Ethics*
• Seeks to educate and to regulate by announcing a **minimal standard of conduct.** Looks mainly at **due Process**	Extends **beyond the law** to prescribe desirable conduct and articulate **ideas and virtues** to which we should aspire

Because respecting law is an important moral duty, the legal cases have ethical relevance. However, what is legally permitted may not be ethically justifiable in a particular case.

Different Normative Theories of Ethics

Deontological theory Greek: *deonto* = duty → Duty-Based	Teleological theory Greek *telos* = end → Consequent-Based Consequences ⇒ right or wrong
⇒ Obligations and duties in the forms of rules and principles	

What you Understand by the "4 Principle" Approach Towards Ethics?

NONMALEFICENCE
= The obligation to avoid the causation of harm
→ Requires merely the omission of harm-causing activities

BENEFICENCE
= The obligation to provide benefits and to balance benefits against risks
→ Requires positive steps to help others

RESPECT FOR AUTONOMY
= The obligation to respect the decision-making capacities of autonomous activities
→ Rooted in the liberal western tradition of the importance of individual freedom, both for political life and for personal development

JUSTICE
= Obligations of fairness in the distribution of benefits and risks

Table 8.2: Difference between clinical ethics *vs* research ethics

	Clinical Ethics	*Research Ethics*
Relationship	Doctor-patient	Researcher-patient → competing and conflicting interests
Primary Objective	Fiduciary→therapeutic effect to benefit patient	Generalized knowledge to benefit society

(Contd.)

(Contd.)

Non-Maleficence	"Above all, do no harm."	Risk of harm always exists → risk-benefit ratio
Intervention	Proven or established treatments	Experimental treatment → clinical equipoise
Consent	Implied and verbal consent applies except for high risk treatment	Full informed consent process and document except for minimal risk research

Why must Clinical Research Be Ethical?

- Clinical research involves many participants
- As a result, there exists the potential for exploitation of research participants.

What are Ethics of Clinical Research?

- Ethical requirements in clinical research to:
- Minimize the possibility of exploitation
- Ensure that subjects' rights and welfare are respected while contributing to the generation of knowledge

Different Codes and Guidelines of Clinical Research

- Nuremberg Code (1949)
- Declaration of Helsinki (1964, 75, 83, 89, 96, 2000)
- The Belmont Report (1979)—National Commission for the Protection of Human Subjects of Biomedical and Behavioral Research
- CIOMS (Council for International Organizations of Medical Sciences)/WHO International Ethical Guidelines for Biomedical Research Involving Human Subjects (1993, 2002)
- ICH/GCP—International Conference on Harmonization—Good Clinical Practice (1996)
- **NC**—Condemns atrocities of the Nazi physicians and focused on (1) need for consent (2) favorable risk benefit ratio makes no mention of fair subject selection or independent review.
- **DH**—Focuses on the deficiency of NC. Also emphasizes a distinction between therapeutic and non-therapeutic research.
- **BR**—Provided broad principles in response to US search scandals such as Tuskegee and Willowbrook.
- **CIOMS**—Intended to apply DH in developing countries large scale trial of vaccines and drugs. 1949-WHO and UNISCO.

Ethical Framework: Existing Guidance

- Finally some tensions, if not outright contradictions, exist among the provisions of various guidelines.
- Hence requirement for a systematic, coherent, universally applicable framework

Ethical Framework: 7 Principles

- Valuable scientific question

- Valid scientific methodology
- Fair subject methodology
- Favorable risk-benefit evaluation
- Independent review
- Informed consent
- Respect for enrolled subjects

Source: Emanuel E et. al., Journal of the American Medical Association 2000; 283(20): 2701-11

1. Valuable Scientific Question

- Question should contribute to overall health and well-being.
- Results should be shared.

2. Valid Methodology

- Based on appropriate laboratory and animal studies
- Design should answer scientific question
  - Include sufficient numbers, the requisite comparison groups, necessary tests, etc.

Feasible Methodology

- Assessment of feasibility must consider
  - The nature of the disease
  - The community in question
  - The resources available for the study
- Study, as designed, is likely to be completed

3. Equitable Participant Selection

- Fair distribution of risks and potential benefits within and across communities
- No participant excluded without a good scientific or ethical reason

4. Research as Risk or Benefit?

Subjects need protection
Subjects need access
Balance of Risks and Benefits required

4.a. Acceptable Risk/Benefit Ratio

Non-maleficence and Beneficence
- Weigh risks against potential benefits
- Ensure potential benefits clearly outweigh risks
- Minimize risks
  - Use qualified research team
  - Eliminate duplicative procedures
- Maximize potential benefits
  - Maximize scientific information
  - Provide participants clinically relevant information

5. Independent Review

Independent Review of clinical research ensures the public that:
- Investigator bias has not distorted the approach
- Ethical requirements have been fulfilled
- Subjects will not be exploited

5.a. Independent Review

- Independent Committee needs:
  - Scientific, cultural, and ethical expertise
  - Authority to modify or stop the study
- Committee should provide initial and ongoing assurance that ethical principles are met.

5.b. AIM of IRB Review-45 CFR 46, Sub Part A

- Minimize risks
- Risks dare justified by anticipated benefits, if any, to the subjects or the importance of the knowledge to be gained
- To check that
  - The subjects are selected and treated fairly
  - Informed consent is adequate

5.c. Composition of IRB/EC

- At least 7 members with
  - Chairperson (outside the institution)
  - Member Secretary
- Protocol review quorum of 5 members at least—
  - Basic medical scientist (pharmacologist preferably)
  - Clinicians
  - Legal expert
  - Social scientist/Representative of non-governmental voluntary agency/philosopher/ethicist/theologian or a similar person
  - Lay person from the community

5.d. Ethics Committee: Ethical Responsibilities

- Assure the safety and welfare of participant subjects
- Approve the protocol and consent form
- Hold periodic meetings
- Maintain records
- Approve conduct of trial
- Review safety reports
- Verify the provisions for injuries
- Review and approve payments to participants
- Interrupt or cancel the trial in case of risk

6. Informed and Voluntary Consent

- All participants should understand

- Their medical and personal situation
- The purpose, methods, risks, potential benefits, and alternatives to the research
- All participants should make a voluntary decision whether to enroll

6.a. Informed Consent

Respect for Persons

- The voluntary consent of the human subject is absolutely essential. (Nuremberg Code)
- For all biomedical research involving human subjects, the investigator must obtain the informed consent of the prospective subject... or authorized representative. (CIOMS guidelines)

6.b. Informed Consent

- Consent process: information, comprehension, and voluntaries
- The subjects should be given the opportunity to choose what shall or shall not happen to them. (The Belmont Report)

6.c. What if Some Individuals are Unable to Consent?

- Avoid enrolling individuals who are unable to consent
- Have safeguards in place when there is a good scientific reason to enroll them
  - Proxy decision maker
  - Ascent

7. Respect for Enrolled Participants

- During the course of the experiment the human subject should be at liberty to bring the experiment to an end... Nuremberg Code... Every precaution should be taken to respect the privacy of the subject, confidentiality of the subject's information, and to minimize the impact of the study on physical and mental integrity and on the personality of the subject. (Helsinki 2000)

7.a. How to Respect Enrolled Participants?

- Protect confidentiality/privacy
- Give participant's new information when possible

Essential Elements of Ethical Research

- Independent Review
- Informed Consent
- Audit
- Balancing Principles
- Clinical Equipoise
- Randomization
- Choice of control

1. Audit

- ICH GCP 1.6 - - Definition
- A systematic and independent examination of trial-related activities and documents

- To determine whether the evaluated trial-related activities were conducted, and the data were recorded, analyzed and accurately reported according to the protocol, sponsor's SOP, GCP and the applicable regulatory requirement(s)

1.a. Type of Audits

- Routine inspections
- To assure compliance with sponsor, federal and local regulations
- "For cause" Auditing group has evidence or suspects non-compliance with some aspect of the clinical trial requirements

1.b. Audits

- Who conducts?
- Sponsor, regulatory department
- Representatives from
- International regulatory authorities
- Local regulatory authorities
- When audits occur?
- During the trial
- After the trial has been completed

1.c. Common Audit Findings

- Protocol non-compliance
- Inadequate source documents
- Inadequate investigational product(s) records
- Informed consent issues

2. Balancing Principles

- A rigorous design <-> maximizing benefits/minimizing harms
- Equipoise
- Randomization

2.a. Clinical Equipoise

"Genuine uncertainty within the scientific community..." about the comparative merits of intervention 'A' and 'B'. (Freedman, 1987)
- Provides a clear moral foundation to the requirement that the health care of subjects is not disadvantaged by research participation

2.b. Randomization

- Random assignment
- No individualization
- No preferences
- Do participants understand random assignment?
- Select a design, e.g. single blind, double blind
- Example: Randomized controlled trials

3. *Choice of Control*

- "The Benefits, risks, burdens and effectiveness of a new method should be tested against those of the best current prophylactic, diagnostic, and therapeutic methods." (Helsinki 2000)
- Balance the need to answer the valuable question in a scientifically rigorous way, with consideration of risks and benefits.

Current Issues which Needs to be Answered?

- Is it acceptable to pay subjects to enroll in research?
- Is there a maximum threshold of net risks to which subjects may be exposed?
- Is it ethical to expose individuals who cannot consent to research risks? Kids?

Other Issues?

- Conflicts of interest: is it acceptable for investigators to have a monetary stake in their research?
- Should there be independent monitors of research?
- Issues in research in developing countries: Access post trial, relevance, standard of care.

Ethics can be explained through the Famous Poem of "The Blind men and the Elephant"

- By John Godfrey Saxe (1816–1887)
- Each man, after experiencing the elephant, is convinced that his opinion was the only correct one, leading to inability to see the bigger picture.
- Like the elephant, scope of ethics cannot be easily explained because the very definition of "ethics" is much beyond what we understand.
- Fundamental accepted principle of modern clinical research ethics is based on a very simple goal—that one cannot inflict harm on research participants for the sake of benefit to future patients.

CONCLUSIONS

A challenging balance
Justice, Risk and Consent
"If a community is to bear the risk of research, it must also reap future benefits".

Links to More Information

- http://www.wma.net
- http://cme.nci.nih.gov
- http://ohrp.osophs.dhhs.gov
- http://ohsr.od.nih.gov/_
- http://www.coims.ch
- http://www/fda.gov

Ethical Issues in Clinical Trials

2

Arun Bhatt

"There is but one law for all; namely the law which governs all laws – the law of our Creator, the law of humanity, justice, equity; the law of nature and of nations."

– Edmund Burke

INTRODUCTION

Ethics concerns all aspects of human society and scientific research is no exception. The larger debate – science *vs* society – acquires a unique dimension in relation to drug research. Clinical trials, which form the backbone of drug development, pose a special challenge to ethicists, as the potential clinical trial subject, who is likely to benefit from a marketed drug, is also at the risk of adverse events of the investigational product (IP). However, unless the human subjects participate in the clinical trial, the benefit risk ratio of an IP cannot be assessed and the IP cannot be developed into a useful therapy. This ethical dilemma continues to challenge all the stake holders - pharma industry, investigators, regulators, and ethics committees (EC) — as novel therapies based on new disciplines, e.g. genomics provide potential new drugs. This article reviews some of the ethical issues in the clinical trials and the current approaches to cope with them.

Ethical Issues

The ethical issues in clinical trials cover the whole spectrum of trial conduct. Some of the issues are:

- Why is the clinical trial required?
- Is the available information on investigational product IP adequate to assess its benefits and risks?
- What are the potential benefits of the IP for the subjects?
- Does IP have any potential advantages over existing standard treatment?
- What are the potential risks of IP for the subjects?
- Is the benefit risk ratio of IP acceptable?
- Is the research methodology scientifically valid?
- What are the consequences of the subject receiving a placebo?
- What are the physical risks/inconveniences of trial procedures/lab tests for the subjects?
- Are there any economic consequences for the subject?
- Is the investigator competent to conduct the trial?
- Is the subject informed about the risks and benefits of participating in the trial?
- What are arrangements of treating the subject who suffer from medical injury/adverse event?
- What is the financial compensation for the subject who suffers from an adverse event/injury?
- Does the patient have the right to withdraw from the trial?
- Is there a risk of discovering sensitive information, e.g. HIV status, genetic profile?

- How will the confidentiality of the subject's identity and medical information be guarded?
- Is the investigational therapy relevant to the country/population?
- Will the patients who take part in the trial, get free supplies of the IP after the trial is over?
- When will the trial results be published?
- What will be impact of trial results on the society?

These ethical issues have evolved over last several decades and have been the subject of several codes and guidelines.

Evolution of Ethics (Table 8.3)

The Second World War (1939-45) crimes against the innocent human beings brought in to highlight the need for a globally relevant ethical code of research conduct. The first International Statement on the ethics of medical research — the **Nuremberg Code** was developed in 1947.[1]

These efforts were reinforced by the World Medical Association which formulated **Declaration of Helsinki** in 1964[2] (Table 8.5). This declaration discusses the responsibilities of medical practitioners in clinical research and is revised regularly in line with evolving ethical requirements the US National Commission for the Protection of Human Subjects of Biomedical and Behavioral Research released the **Belmont Report** in 1979 which covers Ethical Principles and Guidelines for the Protection of Human Subjects of Research.[3] These codes and guidelines are at the root of International Conference on Harmonisation (ICH) on guidelines of **Good Clinical Practice (GCP)** in 1996.[4] (Tables 8.6, 8.7)

Table 8.3: Evolution of ethical guidelines

• 1947	:	Nuremberg code
• 1964	:	Declaration of Helsinki
• 1979	:	Belmont Report
• 1996	:	ICH guidelines
• 2000	:	ICMR guidelines
• 2001	:	Indian GCP guidelines
• 2005	:	Revision of Schedule Y

Table 8.4: Nuremberg code

- Voluntary consent of the human subject
- Anticipate scientific benefits
- Benefits outweigh risks
- Experiment based on adequate animal experimentation
- Avoid all unnecessary physical and mental suffering and injury
- Avoid any experiment where there is a high chance of death or disabling injury
- Protection of the experimental subject from harm
- Scientifically qualified investigators
- Subject at liberty to stop participation
- Investigator will stop experiment if there is likelihood of harm to the subject by continuing the experiment

Table 8.5: Declaration of Helsinki

- Duty of physician to protect the life, health, privacy and dignity of the human subject
- Review of proposed research by independent ethics committee
- Medical research involving human subjects only by scientifically qualified persons and under the supervision of a clinically competent medical person
- Favourable benefit risk ratio
- Physician to obtain the subject's freely-given consent, preferably in writing
- Stress on publication of results — negative or positive
- Effectiveness of a new method to be compared against best current prophylactic, diagnostic, and therapeutic methods
- At the conclusion of the study, every participating patient assured of access to the best proven prophylactic, diagnostic and therapeutic methods identified by the study.

Table 8.6: Principles of ICH-GCP

- Ethical principles - Declaration of Helsinki, GCP and regulatory requirements
- Benefits *vs* Risks
- Safety of subjects *vs* interest of science/society
- Adequacy of non-clinical and clinical information
- Clinical trials scientifically sound and described in clear, detailed protocol
- Compliance with protocol that has received prior approval of EC/IRB
- Medical care responsibility of qualified physician/dentist
- Each individual involved in trial qualified by education, training and experience
- Informed consent freely given
- Information recorded, handled, stored for accurate reporting, information and verification
- Protection of subject's confidentiality
- Investigational products manufactured, stored and handled as per GMP
- Systems with procedures for quality assurance

Table 8.7: Indian Council of Medical Research Guidelines/Indian GCP – Principles

- Essentiality of research
- Voluntariness of participation — informed consent
- Non-exploitation
- Privacy and confidentiality
- Precaution and risk minimization
- Professional competence of researcher
- Accountability and transparency
- Maximization of public interest and distributive justice
- Institutional arrangements
- Public domain
- Totality of responsibility
- Compliance to guidelines

In 1982 the Indian Council of Medical Research prepared a **Policy Statement on Ethical Considerations involved in Research on Human Subjects** for the benefit of all those involved in clinical research in India. In 1982, the World Health Organisation (WHO) and the CIOMS issued the **Proposed International Guidelines for Biomedical Research involving Human Subjects.** The Indian guidelines—**ICMR Ethical Guidelines for Biomedical Research on Human Subjects** 2000 [5] and **Central Drugs Control Standard Organisation (CDSCO) GCP guidelines** 2001[6]—are based on these Indian and global ethical norms.

The main tenets of these codes and guidelines are:

- Autonomy, or respect for persons
- Beneficence, or do good
- Justice
- Non-maleficence, or do no harm

Besides, they also cover the principles and practices for ethical conduct during clinical research (Tables 8.2 to 8.4).

GCP Guidelines – Current Ethical Norm

Good Clinical Practice (GCP) is an international ethical and scientific quality standard for designing, conducting, recording and reporting trials that involve the participation of human subjects. Compliance with this standard provides public assurance that the rights, safety and well-being of trial subjects are protected, and that the clinical trial data are credible.[5, 6]

GCP guidelines provide a process and show the path to managing ethical issues in a clinical trial.

GCP is a shared ethical responsibility for all the stake holders and the guidelines prescribe the responsibilities for each stake holder–EC, investigator and sponsor

An EC has to safeguard the rights, safety, and well-being of all trial subjects. The basic responsibility of an IEC is to ensure a competent review of all ethical aspects of the project proposals received and execute the same free from any bias and influence that could affect their objectivity.

The investigator has to be aware of, and has to comply with, GCP and the applicable regulatory requirements and has to act according to the Declaration of Helsinki. He is responsible for obtaining informed consent, and guarding the health and safety of the trial subjects.

The sponsor is responsible for implementing and maintaining quality assurance and quality control systems with written SOPs to ensure that trials are conducted and data are generated, documented (recorded), and reported in compliance with the protocol, GCP, and the applicable regulatory requirements. The sponsor is also responsible for organising monitoring of the clinical trials, the main purpose of which is to verify that the rights and well-being of human subjects are protected. Besides, the sponsor has to agree, before the research begins, to provide compensation for any serious physical or mental injury for which subjects are entitled to compensation or agree to provide insurance coverage for an unforeseen injury whenever possible.

CONCLUSION

Clinical trials involve human beings as experimental subjects and raise many ethical issues. The Nuremberg Code, Declaration of Helsinki, and GCP guidelines recommend the global norms of ethical conduct. These guiding principles encompass (1) assessment of potential value of information from research (2) scientific rigor in planning (3) fair subject selection (4) favourable risk-benefit ratio

(5) independent review by EC (6) informed consent (7) respect for enrolled subjects (8) protection of the subjects' privacy (9) opportunity for the subject to withdraw and (10) assurance of protecting their well-being.[7] It is mandatory to fulfil all these requirements to ensure that the conduct of clinical trial is ethical.

REFERENCES

1. Trials of War Criminals before the Nuremberg Military Tribunals under Control Council Law No. 10, Vol. 2, pp. 181–182. Washington, D.C.: U.S. Government Printing Office, 1949

2. World Medical Association Declaration of Helsinki Ethical Principles For Medical Research Involving Human Subjects WMA General Assembly, Tokyo 2004

3. The National Commission for the Protection of Human Subjects of Biomedical and Behavioral Research. The Belmont Report, Ethical Principles and Guidelines for the Protection of Human Subjects of Research. Washington, DC: Department of Health, Education and Welfare; 1979

4. International Conference on Harmonisation. Note for Guidance on Good Clinical Practice. ICH Topic E 6. Guideline for Good Clinical Practice. London, United Kingdom: The European Agency for the Evaluation of Medicinal Products; 1996

5. Indian Council of Medical Research Ethical Guidelines for Biomedical Research on Human Subjects New Delhi 2000

6. Central Drugs Standard Control Organisation (CDSCO) Good Clinical Practices for Clinical Research in India 2001

7. Emanuel EJ, Wendler D, Grady C What Makes Clinical Research Ethical? JAMA 283:2701-2711 2000

Chapter 9

Method of Sample Preparation of Some Common Drugs from Biological Fluids

Vivek R. Dhole

HPLC system has several facilities which can be utilised to detect the drugs in the biological materials, such as blood, urine, etc. Selective detection of drugs relative to the matrix is achieved by selecting the suitable stationary phase or even the composition of the mobile phase can be altered to achieve such separation. The sample preparation involves several factors, including the nature of the sample blood, urine, etc., the condition of the sample, and concentration level of the drug. Interference from the matrix components is maximum when the concentration of the drug is very low and special sample preparation is often required. Conditions of the sample also affects such assay, e.g. recoveries from fresh blood and the haemolysed one may not be similar by the same sample preparation method.

FILTRATION METHODS

The most common method for cleaning the sample is by filtration, either by the filter paper or sintered glass crucible. The filter itself is first washed with the solvent. The solvents are selected in such a way so as to dissolve the maximum possible amount of the solute of interest. However, if solutes of interest are present at a very low concentrations, i.e., in ppm levels, a significant amount of them may be lost because of their adsorption on the matrix solid material that is being removed from the sample by way of filtration. Such problems of adsorption are considerably reduced if the contaminating solid material is removed by centrifugation.

PRECIPITATION AND CENTRIFUGATION TECHNIQUES

Drug which is physically or chemically bound to the surface of the proteins, must be released, then the protein is precipitated to leave the drug in aqueous solution. The protein may be degraded by strong acids or enzymes or precipitated by some chemicals like ammonium sulphate or removed by ultrafiltration. But some drugs are susceptible to protein degradation methods and sometimes precipitation and ultrafiltration can lead to losses because of their binding to the proteins. A single procedure cannot work for recovery of all types of drugs from different types of substrate materials. Direct injections of deproteinised solutions are made and analysed on HPLC system by using the polar mobile phase. The biological fluid is mixed and shaken with methanol or acetonitrile and centrifuged to remove the precipitated proteins and the supernatant liquid is used for injection. The proteins are separated out before injection to protect the sample valve and analytical column from irreversible contamination and clogging. Urine can be similarly treated to remove the salts. The centrifugation method, though requires a special micro centrifuge apparatus, has several merits over the other purification methods. Firstly, there is no filter device on which trace components of the sample can be lost due to adsorption, secondly, the sample volume is not changed during the solid removal. Small glass centrifuge tubes are used but if strongly polar trace materials/solutes are present, they may be adsorbed by the polar hydroxyl groups on the wall of the glass tubes, in such cases the tube wall can be deactivated by reacting the surface hydroxyl groups with appropriate alkyl silane groups.

In the centrifugation method, nature of the matrix, nature of the solutes, degree of adsorption of the solute with the matrix, choice of suitable solvent for the maximum solubility of the solute in the solvent play the major role in achieving the maximum per cent recovery of the solute from the matrix.

EXTRACTION AND CONCENTRATION TECHNIQUE

Because of the limited detector sensitivity, there is very often a need of extracting and then concentrating the analyte solution while determining the traces, especially in the biomedical, forensic and environmental samples. Solvent extraction is the most popular approach, as several parameters can be modified to optimise the extent of extraction. Such modifications include changing the polarity of the organic solvent, the pH and ionic nature and strength of the aqueous phase and use of ion pairing agents. After extracting the sample by suitable solvent the organic extract may be directly injected into the column after using the centrifugation or filtration methods or the analyte solution is further concentrated by evaporation, where the solutes are relatively, sufficiently non-volatile compared to the solvents in which they are dissolved. For the oxidisable compounds the evaporation can be carried out in presence of nitrogen and thermally labile compounds also have to be concentrated by evaporation below the thermal decomposition temperature.

LYOPHILISATION

It is a similar technique but it is evaporation at reduced temperature under vacuum. Some aqueous samples can be frozen and the vapor pressure of the ice is sufficient to produce a relatively faster rate of evaporation. Also, where the analytes have sufficiently high vapor pressures at room temperatures, to cause loss of solute by normal evaporation procedures, the Lyophilisation method is used. This method is gentler than the evaporation and hence is being used for the samples of biological origin and the thermally labile analytes and for substances like proteins which denature easily. Special equipments are available for Lyophilisation.

UTILITY OF GUARD COLUMNS

A short guard column is generally introduced between the injector and the analytical column. It is packed with the same material as the analytical column with a larger particle size to minimize the pressure drop and is replaced after some specific duration due to contamination. The ratio of guard column volume to analytical column volume should be around 1 : 20, which keeps band broadening to the minimum, while maintaining sufficient capacity to retain the impurities. Usually the guard column is introduced to increase the life of the analytical column by removing the particulate matter and impurities from the solvent components that bind irreversibly to the stationary phase. Also, in liquid chromatography, the guard column serves to saturate the mobile phase with the stationary phase so that the losses of the solvent from the analytical column are minimised. Thus, the guard column protects the more expensive analytical column. But such a device introduces an extra column volume in the chromatographic system, causing peak dispersion and thus impair resolution where just a marginal level of resolution is achieved with the selected phase system.

SOLID PHASE EXTRACTION (SPE) PROCEDURE

The Solid Phase Extraction (SPE) Fig. 9.1 method involves the use of the short inert plastic cartridge (tube) packed with an adsorbent, usually a reversed phase or an ion exchange resin. The particle size is usually larger than that used in the LC analytical column to avoid the pressure drop and to ensure the reasonable permeability. Depending upon the type of application, a wide variety of materials can be chosen as the adsorbent, which may range from silica gel, reverse phase material, ion exchange resins to affinity packings.

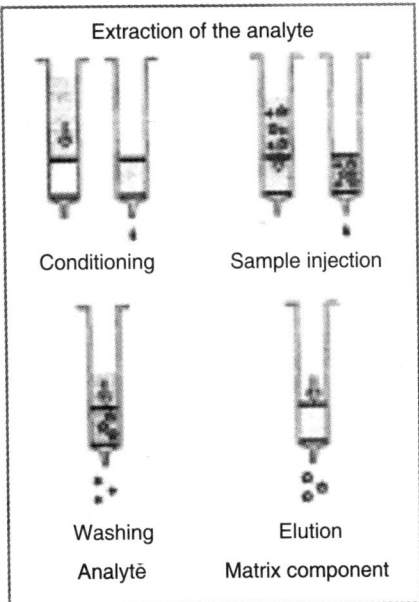

Fig. 9.1. SPE Technique

Thus, solid phase extraction is essentially an extraction process which comprises a solid and a liquid phase. The components of interest and the matrix interference are in the liquid phase. SPE is based on the principle that the components of interest, mainly organic compounds, are mainly retained on the solid adsorbent placed in a disposable cartridge. The interfering components and solvent molecules (matrix) are not retained; and are washed with the suitable solvent. The remaining interfering components are removed from the adsorbent by elution with other suitable solvent. Finally, the analyte is removed from the adsorbent by elution with the suitable solvent, or mobile phase.

The main objectives of SPE are removal of interfering matrix components and selective separation and concentration of analytes. Enrichment can increase the detection sensitivity of the analytes by the factor of 100 to 5000. Such an enrichment is useful for trace level qualitative and quantitative analysis of analytes and also the separation from interfering matrix components.

SPE involves Four Steps

(*a*) **Conditioning of the sorbent:** Usually effected by passing the solvent prior to sample injection, so that the sorbent in the SPE cartridge can interact with the sample. This process is also called as salvation.

(*b*) **Sample injection:** After conditioning the adsorbent bed should not run dry, otherwise solvation is non-effective. Then, the sample solution is forced through the sorbent of the cartridge at about 3 ml/min flow rate. The components of interest (analytes) are adsorbed by the sorbent.

(*c*) **Washing of the adsorbent:** It is being achieved by using some solvents to remove undesired matrix components from the cartridge.

(*d*) **Elution:** Elution is effected by selectively desorbing the compounds of interest from the sorbent and collecting the cartridge effluent.

SPE has become a safe, powerful and fast means of sample preparation having applications in the environmental, pharmaceutical, food, forensic and biochemical analyses, e.g. isolation of analytes such as PCBs, pesticides, PAHs, drugs, vitamins and dyes from matrices such as water, soil, tablets, blood, urine, food stuffs, vegetables and fruits is effected.

Automatic Solid Phase Extraction System

A typical of such system comprises auto sampler, SPE pump, SPE cartridges, switching valves, separate pumps for binary high pressure gradient HPLC system, an analytical HPLC column and suitable detector (usually UV detector). A typical of such system is manufactured as 'UNEXAS' system by M/s. Knauer, Germany, which is being marketed in India by M/s. Chemito Instruments Pvt. Ltd., Mumbai (Fig. 9.2).

UNEXAS

Universal Sample Extraction and Separation

Online Sample Purification and Enrichment is excellently achieved with UNEXAS system.

Benefits of on-line SPE

Full automation: No user intervention between elution from SPE and introduction to HPLC system.

Excellent performance/reduced cost: Elimination of elute collection, evaporation, reconstitution and injection improves precision and sensitivity; saves also time and solvent.

Closed system: Samples are protected against contamination, light and air.

UNEXAS Hardware

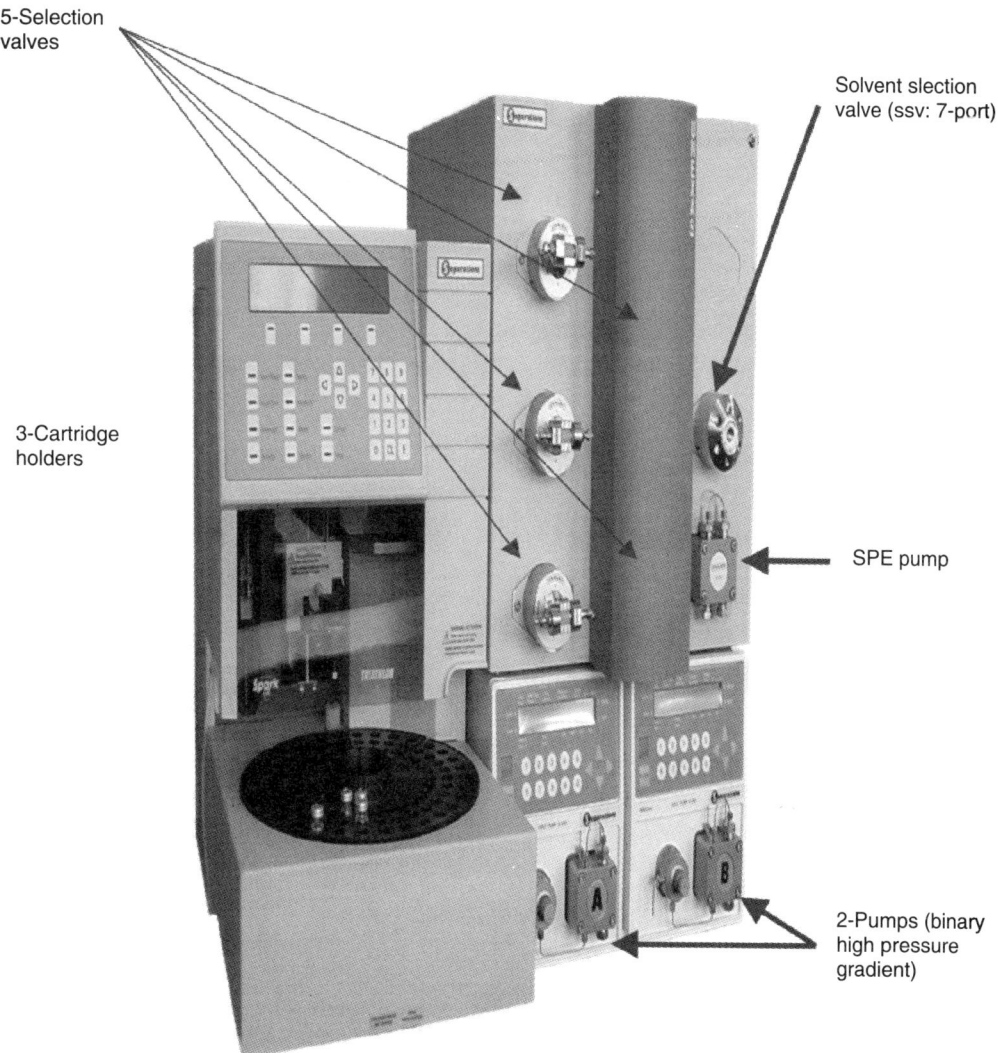

Fig. 9.2. UNEXAS hardware

SPE (4 steps): (Fig. 9.3)

- Activation and conditioning of the SPE cartridges
- Loading of the sample in loop and then to SPE cartridges
- Washing the cartridges
- Elution of the cartridges directly to the HPLC column

HPLC: Start of the Gradient for the Separation and Data Collection

A. Activation and conditioning of the cartridge A:

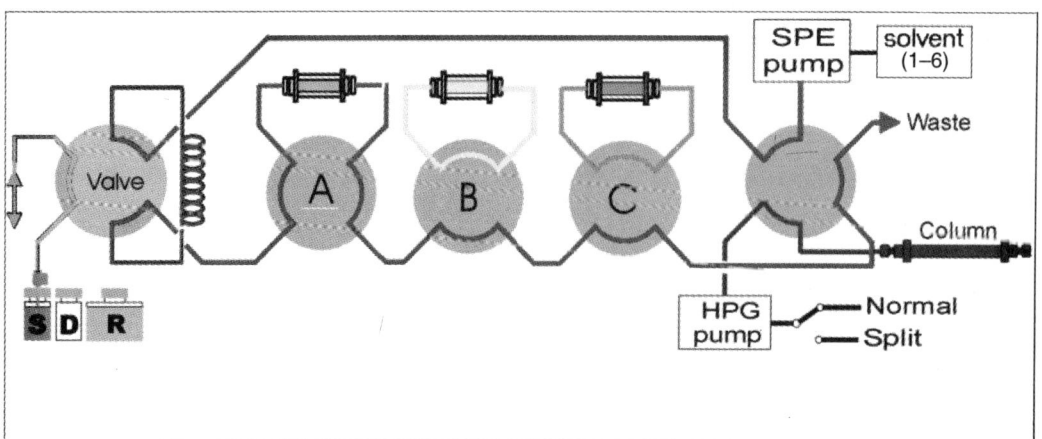

B. First loading of the sample into sample loop and then sample loading to SPE cartridge A:

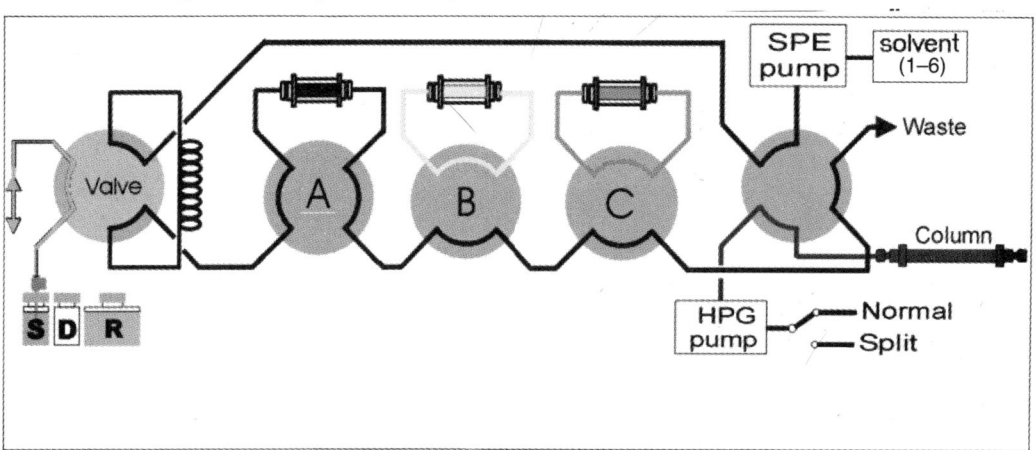

C. Sample washing on the cartridge A with one of the solvents (1–6):

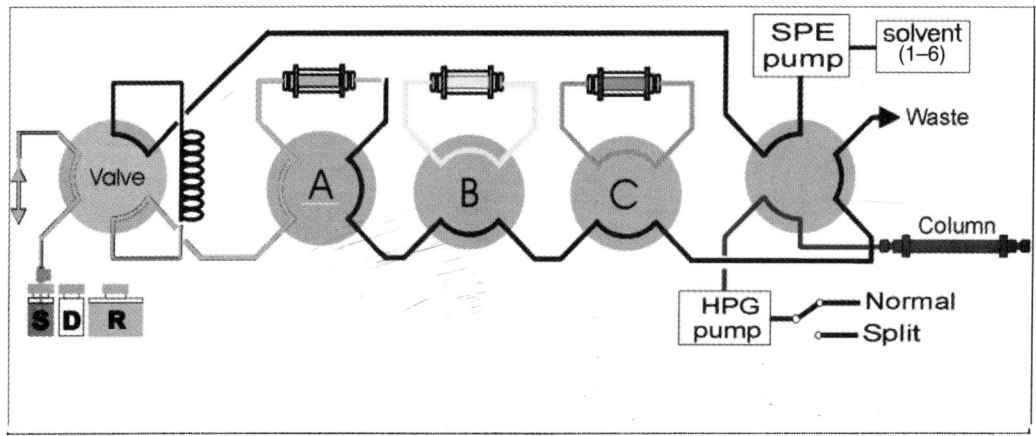

D. Online elution of the sample from cartridge with mobile phase to the HPLC column:

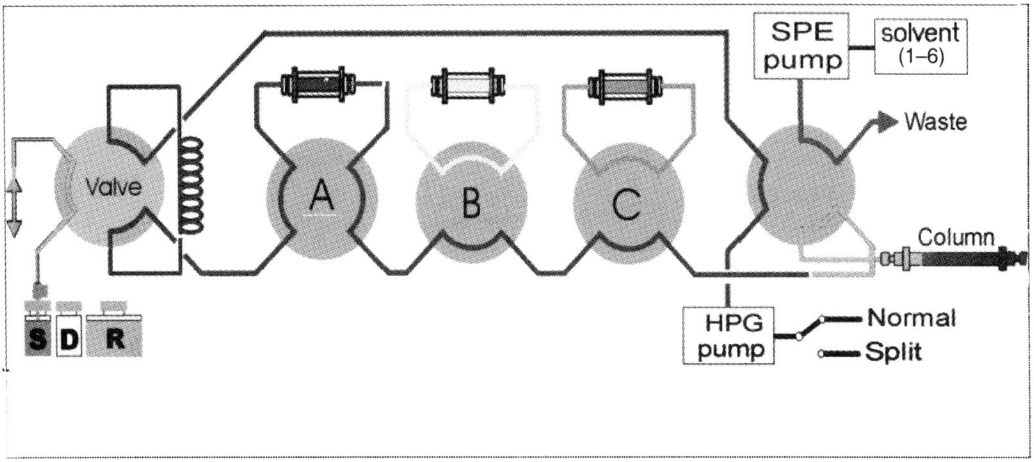

Fig. 9.3. Different steps of SPE

Application Areas for On-line SPE-HPLC:

- Environmental-rapid screening for target pollutants in waste or surface water nitrobenzene, phenols, (PAH's, pesticides)
- Clinical–therapeutic drug monitoring
- Pharmaceutical–drugs in serum, plasma, urine (steroids, antidepressants)
- Food and beverage analysis

Benefits of UNEXAS

- Instrument with integrated sampling injection, sample preparation and chromatographic separation
- Extraction and separation with high sampling throughput
- Efficient utilisation of the solvents
- High reproducibility with constant flow rates
- Low sample contamination and minimised carry over due to controlled washing steps
- Easy handling in method development
- Fully automated and controlled by Knauer software

Some Popular and typical examples of SPE reported in the literature are as follows:

1. Tetra hydro cannabinol carboxylic acid from urine
2. Tricyclic antidepressant drugs from blood serum
3. Amphetamine, codeine and morphine from blood
4. Individual components in different groups, e.g. aromatic amines, phenols, PCBs, PAHs and pesticides from water and soil (environmental) samples
5. Catecholamines in urine sample
6. Analysis of caffeine in cola samples
7. Benzalkonium chloride from waste water
8. Mycotoxins from apple juice

There are several such applications reported on SPE-HPLC analysis.

HPLC Systems for Commonly Used Drugs

HPLC is a very popular technique for the analysis of various classes of drugs in pharma industries. They can be analysed as such or after extraction from blood, plasma or tissue samples, after using some of the clean up steps as described earlier. The detection of these drugs are usually done by a UV detector or by using diode array or fluorescence detector. Some common examples are given in Table 9.1.

Table 9.1: HPLC analytical data

Drug	Column	Mobile Phase	Detection
Amphetamines and other stimulants	C-18	0.2 m of phosphoric acid and 0.1 m of diethyl amine in 10% MeOH	UV at 250 nm
Antihistamines	Silica	Methanolic amn. Perchlorate (10 mM, pH=6.7)	UV at 254 nm
Barbiturates	C-18	Methanol: 0.1 M sod. dihydrogen phosphate (40:60)	UV at 216 nm
Benzodiazepines	C-18	Methanol: Water: phosphate buffer (55:25:20)	UV at 240 nm
Pencillins	C-18	Methanol/Water 1% $NaHCO_3$ 45:55:0.8	UV at 220 nm
Sodium Ampicillin Sodium Oxacillin Sodium Cloxacillin Sodium Flucloxacillin			
Analgesics Propoxyphene Acetaminophen Codeine	C-18	Acetonitrile/0.05 M KH_2PO_4 Containing 0.02% Triethylamine 40:60: pH – 3.0	UV at 254 nm
Antibiotics Chloramphenicol and its Metabolite	C-8	Acetonitrile/Methanol 20 mM H_3PO_4 Containing 0.02% Triethylamine 6:20:74	UV at 254 nm
Antibacterials Trimethoprim Sulfamethoxazole Ciprofloxacin	C-18	0.1% Triethylamine in 20% Acetonitrile pH-9 Phosphate Buffer/Acetonitrile/Methanol 81:5:14	UV at 254 nm Fluorescence EX. 270 nm EM. 440 nm
Hydrocortisone	C-18	Sodium Acetate Buffer/(0.05 ml/litre pH 8) Acetonitrile 77:23	UV at 254 nm
Ibuprofen	C-18	Acetonitrile/Water/Glacial Acetic Acid 45:55:0:32	UV at 240 nm
Theophylline Caffeine Chloramphenicol Phenytoin	C-8	Acetonitrile/Water 20:80	UV at 208 nm

There are several such HPLC methods reported for the analysis of drugs in pharma and biomedical applications, and day by day field of HPLC analytical technique is growing enormously.

Chapter 10

Bioequivalence Study under the Purview of Clinical Trial

Uttam Kumar Mandal
T.K. Pal

INTRODUCTION

Bioequivalence is defined as the absence of a significant difference in the rate and extent to which the active ingredient or active moiety in pharmaceutical dosage form becomes available at the site of drug action when administered at the same molar dose under similar conditions in an appropriately designed study. BE documentation can be useful during the IND and NDA period to establish links between (1) early and late clinical trial formulations; (2) formulations used in clinical trial and stability studies, if different; (3) clinical trial formulations and to-be-marketed drug product. BE studies are critical component in the postapproval period for certain changes in both NDAs and ANDAs.

DEFINITION OF BIOAVAILABILITY AND BIOEQUIVALENCE

Bioavailability

Bioavailability means the rate and extent to which the active substance or therapeutic moiety is absorbed from a pharmaceutical form and becomes available at the site of action.[1,2]

In the majority of cases substances are intended to exhibit a systemic therapeutic effect, and a more practical definition can then be given, taking into consideration that the substance in the general circulation is in exchange with the substance at the site of action.

Bioavailability is understood to be the extent and the rate to which a substance or its therapeutic moiety is delivered from a pharmaceutical form into the general circulation.

Bioequivalence

Bioequivalence means the absence of a significant difference in the rate and extent to which the active ingredient or active moiety in pharmaceutical equivalents or pharmaceutical alternatives becomes available at the site of drug action when administered at the same molar dose under similar conditions in an appropriately designed study.[1,2]

TYPES OF FORMULATIONS WHERE BIOEQUIVALENCE STUDY IS NEEDED[1,2]

Bioequivalence study should be carried out for the following types of formulations containing new/approved active ingredient:

1. Oral immediate release products with systemic action
2. Oral solutions
3. Non-oral immediate release forms with systemic action
4. Modified release dosage form
5. Fixed combination product
6. Parenteral formulations
7. Gases
8. Locally applied products

Requirements for the demonstration of bioequivalence may vary with this type of product.

Oral Immediate Release Products with Systemic Action

Bioequivalence studies should be performed for all immediate release products intended for systemic action unless, considering all of the following criteria, the applicant can establish that *in vitro* are sufficient to ensure bioequivalence.

As an example *in vitro* data alone would be acceptable if all of the following criteria are fulfilled, as follows:

(*i*) The active substance is known not to require special precautions with respect to precision and accuracy of dosing, e.g., it does not have a narrow therapeutic range;

(*ii*) The pharmacokinetics is characterized by a pre-systemic elimination/first pass metabolism less than 70%; and linear pharmacokinetics within the therapeutic range;

(*iii*) The drug is highly water-soluble, i.e. the amount contained in the highest strength is dissolved in 250 ml of each of three pharmacopoeial buffers within the range oh pH 1–8 at 37°C (preferably at or about pH 1.0, 4.6, 6.8);

(*iv*) The drug is highly permeable in the intestine, i.e. its extent of absorption is greater than 80%. Permeability of a drug substance can be determined by different methods, such as, *in vivo* (e.g. $CaCO_2$ cell cultures) and *in situ*, e.g. intestinal perfusion in animals. The choice of the method has to be justified by the applicant in terms of ability to predict the rate and extent of absorption in humans. Stability of the drug should be documented under various conditions typical for the gastrointestinal tract;

(*v*) The excipients included in the composition of the medicinal product are well established and no interaction with the pharmacokinetics of the active substance is expected.

In case an active substance qualifies for exemption, the recipients comply with criterion (*v*) above, the method of manufacture of the finished product in relation with critical physicochemical properties of the active substance (e.g. particle size, polymorphism) should be adequately addressed and documented in the development pharmaceutics section of the dossier.

Oral Solutions

If the product is an aqueous oral solution at the time of administration containing the active substance in the same concentration and form as a currently approved medicinal product, not containing excipients that may effect gastrointestinal transit or absorption of the active substance, then a bioequivalence study is not required.

In those cases where an oral solution has to be tested against a solid dosage form, e.g., an oral solution is formulated to be equivalent to an existing tablet, a comparative bioavailability study will be required unless an exemption can be justified.

Non-oral Immediate Release Forms with Systemic Action

In general bioequivalence studies are required.

Modified Release Dosage Form

Requirements for bioequivalence studies in accordance with specific guidelines.

Fixed Combination Product

Combination products should be assessed with respect to the bioavailability and bioequivalence of individual active substance either separately or as an existing combination.

Parenteral Formulations

The applicant is not required to submit a bioequivalence study if the product is to be administered as an intravenous solution containing the active ingredient in the same concentration as the currently authorized product.

In the case of other parenteral routes, e.g. intramuscular or subcutaneous, the product must be the same type of solution (aqueous or oily), contain the same concentration of the same active substance and the same or comparable excipients as the medicinal product currently approved for this exemption to apply.

Gases

If the product is a gas for inhalation a bioequivalence study is not required.

Locally Applied Products

For products for local use (after oral, nasal, ocular, dermal, rectal, vaginal, etc.) administration intended to act without systemic absorption the approach to determine bioequivalence based on systemic measurements is not applicable and pharmacodynamic or comparative clinical studies are in principle required.

GUIDELINES ON THE DESIGN OF A SINGLE-DOSE BIOEQUIVALENCE STUDY[1]

(a) Basic Principles

1. An *in vivo* bioavailability or bioequivalence study should be a single-dose comparison of the drug product to be tested and the appropriate reference material conducted in normal adults.
2. The test product and the reference material should be administered to subjects in the fasting state, unless some other approach is more appropriate for valid scientific reasons.

(b) Study Design

1. A single-dose study should be crossover in design, unless a parallel design or other design is more appropriate for valid scientific reasons, and should provide for a drug elimination period.

2. Unless some other approach is appropriate for valid scientific reasons, the drug elimination period should be either:

   (*i*) At least three times the half-life of the active drug ingredient or therapeutic moiety, or its metabolite(s), measured in the blood or urine; or

   (*ii*) At least three times the half-life of decay of the acute pharmacological effect.

(c) Collection of Blood Samples

1. When comparison of the test product and the reference material is to be based on blood concentration-time curves, unless some other approach is more appropriate for valid scientific reasons, blood samples should be taken with sufficient frequency to permit an estimate of both:

   (*i*) The peak concentration in the blood of the active drug ingredient or therapeutic moiety, or its metabolite(s), measured; and

   (*ii*) The total area under the curve for a time period at least three times the half-life of the active drug ingredient or therapeutic moiety, or its metabolite(s), measured.

2. In a study comparing oral dosage forms, the sampling times should be identical.

3. In a study comparing an intravenous dosage form and an oral dosage form, the sampling times should be those needed to describe both:

   (*i*) The distribution and elimination phase of the intravenous dosage form;

   (*ii*) The absorption and elimination phase of the oral dosage form.

4. In a study comparing drug delivery systems other than oral or intravenous dosage forms with an appropriate reference standard, the sampling times should be based on valid scientific reasons.

(d) Collection of Urine Samples

When comparison of the test product and the reference material is to be based on cumulative urinary excretion-time curves, unless some other approach is more appropriate for valid scientific reasons, samples of the urine should be collected with sufficient frequency to permit an estimate of the rate and extent of urinary excretion of the active drug ingredient or therapeutic moiety, or its metabolite(s), measured.

(e) Measurement of an Acute Pharmacological Effect

1. When comparison of the test product and the reference material is to be based on acute pharmacological effect-time curves, measurements of this effect should be made with sufficient frequency to permit a reasonable estimate of the total area under the curve for a time period at least three times the half-life of decay of the pharmacological effect, unless some other approach is more appropriate for valid scientific reasons.

2. The use of an acute pharmacological effect to determine bioavailability may further require demonstration of dose-related response. In such a case, bioavailability may be determined by comparison of the dose-response curves as well as the total area under the acute pharmacological effect-time curves for any given dose.

ETHICS REVIEW PROCEDURE

Guidelines as drawn up by the Institutional Review Board are followed with regard to the treatment of human volunteers in the study.[12] These guidelines meet the requirements of the US Code of Federal Regulations (Title 21, Part 56), the Declarations of Helsinki and the Canadian MRC Guidelines. The protocol and the informed consent form are submitted to the appropriate Ethical Committee prior to the initiation of the study. The approval of the Ethical Committee is taken in advance of the study commencement. The study is not started until the approval of the Ethical Committee is received.

INFORMED CONSENT

Before recruitment and enrollment into the study, each prospective candidate is given a full explanation of the study. Once this essential information is provided to the subject and once the physician in charge has the conviction that he understands the implications of participating in the study, the subjects are asked to sign the informed consent form. Table 10.1 shows one blank format of volunteer consent form.

Table 10.1: Bioequivalence/Bioavailability study volunteer consent form

Venue:———— Date: ———— Drug: ———— Dose: ————

1. I .... the undersigned voluntarily agree to take part in the study: titled as: Bioequivalence of ....
   I understand that the investigation will involve the administration of .... X ....
   on .... study days in .... dosing sessions at the interval of .... days.

2. I have been given a full explanation by the member of the study team, of the nature, purpose and likely duration of the study and what I will be expected to do and I have been advised about my discomfort and possible ill effects on my health or well-being which he believes may result.

3. I have been given the opportunity to question the study team, on aspects of the study and have understood the advice and information given as a result.

4. I agree to comply with any instruction given during the study and to cooperate faithfully with the study team, and to tell immediately, if I suffer from any deterioration of any kind in my health or well-being or any unexpected or unusual symptoms, however, they may have arisen.

5. I agree that I will not seek to restrict the use to which the results of the study may be put in particular; I accept that they may be disclosed to regulatory authorities for medicines.

6. I understand that I am free to withdraw from the study at any time without needing to justify my decision.

Signature of the Volunteer: Address: ....
                                                 ....
Date: ....
Signature of the Investigator/Doctor:
Date:
Signature of the Witness:
Date:

SUBJECT SELECTION CRITERIA

Adult, healthy, male, human volunteers with 18 to 40 years of age are selected. The selected volunteers are screened for inclusion in the study within 21 days before the commencement of the study. Demographic data of the volunteers are enlisted according to the Table 10.2.

Table 10.2: Demographic data of 12 volunteers

Vol. No.	Sex	Age	Height (cm)	Weight (kg.)
1	–			
2				
3				
4				
5				
6				
7				
8				
9				
10				
11				
12				
Mean				
S.D.				

Screening Tests

The screening examination was included complete physical and clinical examination, various biochemical and hematological tests. They are:

    (*i*) Complete physical and clinical examination including personal and family history

   (*ii*) Complete hemogram

  (*iii*) LFT (Liver Function Tests) S. Bilirubin, S. Proteins, SGOT, SGPT, Alk. phosphatase

  (*iv*) RFT (Renal Function Tests): BUN, S. Creatinine

   (*v*) S. Proteins

  (*vi*) Blood Sugar (Fasting)

 (*vii*) Virological Tests: HIV Antibody, HBS Ag.

(*viii*) Routine Urine Examination

Inclusion Criteria

   (*i*) 18 to 40 years of age

  (*ii*) Only males

 (*iii*) Weight within 15% of their ideal as of Life Insurance Company's table

 (*iv*) Healthy (eligible after physical, clinical, hematological and biochemical examination)

  (*v*) Normal ECG

 (*vi*) Normal blood pressure and heart rate as measured after resting supine for three minutes. (Normal BP — 100 to 150 mm Hg systolic and 50 to 90 mm Hg diastolic supine, Normal heart rate — 50 to 90 beats per minute).

(*vii*) Ability to communicate well with the investigator

(*viii*) Availability of subject for the entire study period and willingness to adhere to protocol requirements as evidence by written informed consent

(*ix*) Non-smoker.

Exclusion Criteria

(*i*) History of hypersensitivity to the study drug or related products.

(*ii*) Significant history or presence of gastrointestinal, liver or kidney disease, or any other conditions known to interfere with the adsorption, distribution, metabolism or excretion of common medications.

(*iii*) Significant history of asthma, chronic bronchitis or other bronchospastic condition.

(*iv*) Significant history or presence of glaucoma, cardiovascular or haematological disease.

(*v*) Any clinically significant illness during the 4 weeks prior to day 1 of this study.

(*vi*) Maintenance therapy with any drug, or history of drug dependence, alcohol abuse, or serious neurological or psychological disease.

(*vii*) Participation in a clinical trial with an investigation drug within 30 days prior to day 1 of this study.

(*viii*) Use of any systemic medication (including OTC preparations) within 14 days preceding day 1 of this study.

(*ix*) HIV and Australian antigen positive subjects.

(*x*) Clinically relevant abnormal physical and/or clinical findings at the screening.

(*xi*) Abnormal ECG

(*xii*) Loss of greater than 400 ml of blood, in the period 0 to 12 weeks before entry to the study or during the study.

(*xiii*) Serious adverse reaction or hypersensitivity to any drug.

(*xiv*) Inability to communicate or cooperate with the investigator due to language problem, poor mental development or impaired cerebral function.

SUBJECT WITHDRAWAL

If a subject wishes to leave the study at any time, he will be permitted to do so. Every reasonable effort will be made to complete a final assessment.

A subject may withdraw from the study in any of the following circumstances:

(*i*) Serious adverse events

(*ii*) Major violation of the protocol

(*iii*) Withdrawal of the consent

(*iv*) Termination of the study by the sponsor

(*v*) Any systemic illness occurring during the study period requiring intake of other drugs

Any subject discontinuing the trial medication prematurely because of reasons 1 or 5 will be replaced.

DOSING PATTERN

The volunteers are randomized on the previous day of study day 1. In study session I, each volunteer is administered either the test preparation or the reference preparation as single dose on the study day at a fixed time. In study session II, this order is reversed as per the randomization (Table 10.3). For the purpose of accurate sampling time for all samples, study medication is administered at sufficient intervals between 2 subjects. Study medication is given with 240 ml water at room temperature.

Table 10.3: Mode of treatment

Subject No.	Period I	Period II
1	A	B
2	A	B
3	A	B
4	B	A
5	B	A
6	A	B
7	B	A
8	B	A
9	B	A
10	B	A
11	A	B
12	A	B

A – Reference preparation

B – Test preparation

CONCOMITANT MEDICATION

Subjects are informed well in advance not to take any drug for at least 14 days prior to the study. They are specifically reminded not to take cold preparations, vitamins and antacid preparations. In addition, no concomitant medication is permitted during the study period. Each subject is specifically questioned on these points prior to drug administration. The volunteers are also instructed to refrain from consuming alcohol, smoking or any other stimulant drinks, during that period.

SUPPLY OF DRUGS

The test drug in suitable packing and appropriate condition, along with the Certificate of Analysis (COA) and the statement of expiry date is supplied by the sponsor to the Clinical pharmacologist atleast 7 working days prior to the study date. The test drug is stored under the control of the clinical pharmacologist in locked cupboard at ambient temperature unless otherwise advised by the sponsor. Prior to the commencement of the study, the sponsor has to supply a complete Test Material Data Sheet (TMDS) indicating the test material identity, purity, stability, appearance, handling and safety instructions. The TMDS is used as cross-reference to the sponsor's Certificate of Analysis.

BLOOD COLLECTION

All the volunteers are requested to assemble at 6.00 a.m. on the study day 1 of each session, after overnight fasting of at least 10 hrs. Their TPR, BP are recorded and an indwelling intravenous cannula is introduced with strict aseptic precautions in the anticubital vein for blood collection. They are given either of the study preparations (Reference/Test) according to their code nos. with 240 ml of water. The exact clock time is calculated according to the drug administration schedule. The first blood sample ($t = 0$) is collected immediately prior to drug administration. The clock time of all blood draws is recorded and reported for each subject. Any deviation from the sampling schedule is recorded in the subject's sampling time sheet. Sampling time sheets for all subjects are attached in the final report. A total of at least 15 blood samples including at 0 hr are collected from in coded, centrifuge tubes containing EDTA. Blood samples are centrifuged immediately, the plasma are separated into duplicate polypropylene tubes and stored frozen at $-20°$ C. The tubes are labeled with volunteer code number, sampling time and study date (Table 10.4). This code does not reveal the formulation identity.

Table 10.4: Blood sampling schedule

Volunteer Code No.:   Date of Period I of Study:
Bed No.:   Date of Period II of Study:
                                                       Drug Name:
Name of the Volunteer: .... Age:
Address: ....

Sample no.	Interval (hrs)	Actual Timing	Sample Code Phase I	Phase II	Volume of Blood	Menu
1	0		V S 1 P1	V S 1 P2	5 ml	Fruit juice and water
2	1.0		V S 2 P1	V S 2 P2	5 ml	
3	2.0		V S 3 P1	V S 3 P2	5 ml	Breakfast: Bread, banana, boiled egg, milk
4	3.0		V S 4 P1	V S 4 P2	5 ml	
5	4.0		V S 5 P1	V S 5 P2	5 ml	
6	5.0		V S 6 P1	V S 6 P2	5 ml	
7	6.0		V S 7 P1	V S 7 P2	5 ml	Lunch: Rice, dal, vegetables, fish
8	7.0		V S 8 P1	V S 8 P2	5 ml	
9	8.0		V S 9 P1	V S 9 P2	5 ml	
10	10.0		V S 10 P1	V S 10 P2	5 ml	Tiffin: Biscuit, bread, tea, sweet
11	12.0		V S 11 P1	V S 11 P2	5 ml	
12	24.0		V S 12 P1	V S 12 P2	5 ml	
13	48.0		V S 13 P1	V S 13 P2	5 ml	Dinner: Rice, dal, Vegetables, Meat

Attending Supervisors   Clinical Pharmacologist/Doctor   Blood collectors
1...........................   ....   1......................
2...........................   2......................

Chief Investigator   Transporter
....

DIETARY CONTROL

A standardized breakfast, lunch and dinner is served to subjects at 3, 6–8 and 14 hours respectively after drug ingestion. Water is provided *ad libitum* until 1.0 hour predose. Fluid intake is controlled and consistent for the first 3.0 hours following drug administration as follows: drug is given 240 ml of water at room temperature and no fluids except one cup of non-caffeine-containing soft drink is allowed till 3 hours postdose. On the study day, volunteers are permitted normal activities, excluding strenuous exercise.

ANALYSIS OF BLOOD SAMPLES

The concentration of analyte in blood samples is analyzed by HPLC or LC-MS/MS method. The analytical method is validated prior to the start of study according to the ICH and USFDA guidelines.[3,4]

ADVERSE EVENTS

Abnormal symptoms/signs were monitored, during the study period and for one week. No abnormal symptoms were noted during or after the study.

EMERGENCY PROCEDURES

Emergency equipment and drugs should be available in the CPU. Copies of randomization schedule are held by the biostatistician in sealed envelopes. Medical and nursing personnel are engaged during all critical phases of the study. The clinical pharmacologist personally monitors all the events.

QUALITY ASSURANCE

Studies are conducted in accordance with guidance and good clinical research practice in the European Community approved by the CPMP in July 1990.

DOCUMENTATION

All data obtained during the course of the clinical phase of the study are recorded directly and legibly into the Case Record Form in black ink. The clinical pharmacologist prepares the case record forms.

EVALUATION OF PHARMACOKINETIC PARAMETERS

The plasma levels produced by the administration of the studied drug in each volunteer and corrected for the measured content of the dosage form are used to establish the pharmacokinetic profile of test and reference preparations. The plasma drug level profile is presented in tabular and graphical forms. The following pharmacokinetic parameters of test and reference preparations are calculated for each subject.

- C_{max} (Peak plasma concentration)
- t_{max} (Time to maximum plasma concentration)
- $AUC_{(0-t)}$ (The area under plasma concentration time curve 0 to t)
- $AUC_{(0-\mu)}$ (The area under plasma concentration time curve 0 to μ)
- $t_{1/2}$ (Elimination half life)
- K_{el} (Elimination rate constant)

C_{max} and t_{max} are observed values. K_{el} is the elimination rate constant estimated by a linear least-squares regression analysis of the individual concentrations observed as a function of time during the elimination phase. The elimination $t_{1/2}$ is obtained using the following relationship:

$$t_{1/2} = \frac{0.693}{K_{el}}$$

STATISTICAL ANALYSIS

Usual descriptive analyses including the mean and standard deviation (SD) are used for variables such as the height, weight and age. These statistical parameters including coefficient of variance are also used to describe plasma concentrations at each individual time point as well as the pharmacokinetic parameters. Statistical test are applied on untransformed ($C_{max,}$ $AUC_{0-t,}$ AUC_{0-a}) and log-transformed pharmacokinetic data ($C_{max,}$ $AUC_{0-t,}$ AUC_{0-a}). ANOVA of $C_{max,}$ $AUC_{0-t,}$ AUC_{0-a} are subjected to a 2-way ANOVA accounting for subjects, period and treatment.

The design of bioequivalence study is standardized and aimed at separating the treatment (i.e. formulation effect) from other effects. Thus, the study is an open single dose randomized crossover study in healthy male volunteers. With an appropriate washout period between doses, the crossover is ideally suited for comparative bioavailability studies. A washout period of seven half-lives is kept between two treatments, ensuring that less than 1% of drug from the first phase remains in the plasma at the time the second dose is administered.

The typical ANOVA (analysis of variance) for crossover studies is applied to the AUC, $C_{max,}$ and t_{max} data. The ANOVA separates the total sum of squares into four components: subjects, periods, treatments and erreo (residual). The subject sum of squares is separated from the error term, which then represents "intrasubject" variation. The analysis is done using the following equations:

1. Total sum of sqares $(TSS) = \sum X_t^2 - C.T.$

   Where $\sum X_t^2$ is sum of the squared observations.

   $C.T.$ is the correction term

   $$C.T. = \frac{\left(\sum X_t\right)^2}{N_t}$$

   Where $\left(\sum X_t\right)^2$ is the square of sum of all observations.

   N_t is total number of observations

2. Subject sum of squares $(SSS) = \frac{\sum\left(\sum S_t\right)^2}{N_t} - C.T.$

   Where $\sum S_t$ is the sum of observations of a single patient

3. Period sum of squares $(PSS) = \frac{\left(\sum P_1\right)^2 + \left(\sum P_2\right)^2}{12} - C.T.$

   $\sum P_1$ is the sum of observations for Period 1
   $\sum P_2$ is the sum of observations for Period 2

4. Treatment sum of squares $= \dfrac{\left(\sum X_A\right)^2 + \left(\sum X_B\right)^2}{12} - C.T.$

5. Error sum of squares (ESS) = TSS–SSS–PSS– Treatment sum of squares

The degrees of freedom are calculated as follows:

To test for differences between two treatments, an F ratio is formed

F – M.S.S./Error M.S.S.

The F distribution has 1 and 22 degrees of freedom. According to F distribution table an F of 4.35 is needed for significance at the 5% level. Therefore, the two treatments (i.e. the test and reference product) are not significantly different at the 5% level. One typical format for reporting ANOVA results is given in Table 10.5.

Table 10.5: Anova summary format for pharmacokinetic parameter

SOURCE	D.F.	S.S.	M.S.S.	F.	P.
SUBJECTS	11				S/N.S
TREATMENT	1				S/N.S
PERIOD	1				S/N.S
ERROR	10				–
TOTAL	23				–

DF	–	Degree of Freedom
SS	–	Sum of Squares
MSS	–	Mean Sum of Squares
F	–	M.S.S./Error
P	–	Probability
NS	–	Non-significant
S	–	Significant

CONFIDENCE INTERVALS

The analysis of variance is test of the hypothesis of the equality of the AUC_{0-t}, AUC_{0-inf}, C_{max} and t_{max}, for the two formulations. Arguments have been presented that hypothesis testing may not be an appropriate statistical approach to bioequivalence studies. Two different formulations are apt to be different with regard to bioavailability parameters such as AUC_{0-t}, AUC_{0-inf}, and C_{max}. Proposals have been made that a more informative statement about equivalence would be present a "range" of equivalence, a lower and upper limit of the "equivalence" of two formulations. The conventional bioequivalence range for the mean ratio of the variable AUC and C_{max} is 0.8 to 1.25, while the European guideline allows a wider range (0.7 to 1.43) for certain drugs.

CRITERIA FOR BIOEQUIVALENCE

1. AUC_{0-t} of Test formulation/AUC_{0-t} of Reference formulation = 0.8 to 1.25
2. C_{max} of Test formulation/C_{max} of Reference formulation = 0.8 to 1.25

BIOEQUIVALENCE STUDY OF TWO FORMULATIONS CONTAINING 30 MG ARIPIPRAZOLE IN HEALTHY HUMAN VOLUNTEERS: A CASE STUDY

ABSTRACT

Aripiprazole is a new atypical anti-psychotic drug used for the management of schizophrenia, a brain disorder. A simple and sensitive reversed phase high performance liquid chromatography (RP-HPLC) coupled with UV detector (Knauer Germany) set at 215 nm has been used to determine plasma concentration of aripiprazole in healthy male human volunteers. The method has been validated over a linear range of 20–400 ng/ml from plasma. The minimum quantifiable concentration (LOQ) obtained was 20 ng/ml (%CV < 10%). The pharmacokinetic parameters (C_{max}, AUC_{0-t}, $AUC_{0-\infty}$) of this drug have been evaluated by the above method to compare the single oral dose (30 mg) bioavailability of aripiprazole with the reference formulation in 12 healthy male volunteers of two ways, two periods crossover randomized study. Adverse effects leading to postural dizziness and blood pressure lowering have been observed in some of the volunteers although ECG reports confirm the non-significant physiological change. The pharmacokinetic parameters were C_{max} = 118.823 ± 20.764 ng/ml at t_{max} = 3.9583 ± 0.6895 hour, AUC_{0-t} = 4962.6749 ± 1189.5371 ng.hr.ml^{-1}, $AUC_{0-\infty}$ =7266.7500 ± 2146.7847 ng. hr.ml^{-1}, K_{el} = 0.0138334 ± 0.00247 hr^{-1} and $t_{1/2}$ =51.6874 ± 9.804 hr.

INTRODUCTION

Aripiprazole (7-[4-[4-(2, 3- dichloro phenyl)-1- piperazinyl] butoxy]-3, 4- dihydro carbostyril) is a new atypical anti-psychotic drug used for the management of schizophrenia, a brain disorder. It has potent partial agonist activity at dopamine D2 receptor,[5] partial agonist activity at serotonin 5-HT$_{1A}$ receptors[6] and antagonist activity at 5- HT$_{2A}$ receptor.[7] The clinical trial[8] involving pharmacokinetic,[9-13] efficacy and safety evaluations has been revealed that aripiprazole is an effective and well-tolerated drug in the management of schizophrenia. Development of a rapid sensitive and selective method for the determination of aripiprazole in human plasma is essential for understanding the pharmacokinetics of this drug when administered orally. The numbers of published methods for analysis are limited.[14] This paper describes a simple and selective HPLC method with UV-detection to analyze Aripiprazole in human plasma. The aim and objective of the present study were to evaluate the pharmacokinetic parameter for bioequivalence study of tablet aripiprazole 30 mg (aripiprazole tablet from Psycho Remedies, Ludhiana, India) as test formulation and ARIPRA (containing aripiprazole 30 mg) from Ranbaxy SOLUS, New Delhi, India as reference formulation.

THE STUDY

Study design

Adult, healthy, male human volunteers within 18–40 years were selected for the panel of volunteers recruited by CPU (Clinical Pharmacology Unit).

The bioequivalence study of the test preparation was assessed utilizing a typical, two periods randomized, two-way complete crossover design in 12 healthy, male human volunteers. There were two dosing session with a washout period of 15 days between them. All the volunteers are required to participate in two dosing sessions. In each dosing session, volunteers received either of test or reference preparation of tablet aripiprazole 30 mg as a single dose only on the study day as per the randomization code at a fixed time.

Approval from the DCGI (Drugs Controller General of India) as well as clearance from the Institutional Ethical Committee (IEC) was received prior to undertaking this study. The whole study was conducted under the active guidance of clinical pharmacologists.

Blood Collection, Dietary Control and Adverse Events

A total of 15 blood samples were collected from anticubital vein at zero hour (before administration) 0.5, 1, 1.5, 2, 3, 4, 6, 8, 10, 12, 18, 24, 36 and 48 hours in coded, centrifuge tubes containing EDTA. Blood samples were centrifuged immediately, the plasma separated into duplicate polypropylene tubes and stored frozen at $-20°$ C.

A standard breakfast, lunch and dinner was served to subjects at 3, 6–8 and 14 hours respectively after drug ingestion. On the study day, volunteers were permitted normal activities excluding strenuous exercise.

Abnormal symptoms/signs were monitored during the study period and for one week after the study period and if noticed their details were entered in the case report sheets and tabulated at the end of the study.

Stock Solution

Stock solutions of aripiprazole (1 mg/ml) were prepared by dissolving the drug in acetonitrile and stored at $-20°$ C. Appropriate dilution of the stock solutions were prepared by diluting the stock solutions with mobile phase.

Calibration Curves

For calibration curve six different concentrations (20 ng/ml, 50 ng/ml, 100 ng/ml, 150 ng/ml, 200 ng/ml and 400 ng/ml) in plasma were prepared by adding required volume of working solution of analyte to blank plasma. Valdecoxib was taken as Internal Standard and its concentration in plasma was 200 ng/ml. The plasma sample was subjected to the sample preparation procedure and injected onto HPLC. Plasma calibration curve was prepared by taking area ratio of analyte to IS as Y-axis and concentration of analyte (ng/ml) as X-axis.

Chemicals and Reagents Used

Acetonitrile (ACN), HPLC grade water, methylene chloride, KH_2PO_4 and KOH. All the reagents were of HPLC grade.

Chromatographic Conditions

Instrument	:	Knauer HPLC, Germany
Column	:	Hypersil BDS, C18, 150 × 4.6 mm, 5 m particle size, stainless steel.
Mobile Phase	:	10 m. mol phosphate buffer : ACN :: 50 : 50 (v/v)
Flow Rate	:	1 ml/min
Wavelength of detection	:	215 nm
Injector	:	Fixed loop Rheodyne injector system filled with a 20 ml Rhd. Loop.
Integrating Software	:	Eurochrom 2000

Extraction Procedure

1 ml of plasma spiked with aripiprazole raw drug was taken in a stoppered test tube. To this 10 ml of Internal Standard (valdecoxib in ACN) was added and mixed well. This mixture was extracted with

8 ml of methylene chloride followed by shaking for 10 minutes and then centrifuged for three minutes at 3000 RPM. The organic layer was removed in a separate centrifuge tube with cap. The resulting organic layer was evaporated to dryness in water bath in presence of nitrogen atmosphere at 40°C. The residue was reconstituted with 150 ml of dilute H_3PO_4 and the same was injected onto HPLC for chromatographic analysis.

Accuracy, Precision and Freeze Thaw Recovery

Within–run, between–run precision and accuracy as well as Freeze thaw recovery was carried out as per the protocol described in our earlier paper.[15-17]

RESULTS AND DISCUSSION

The described analytical method used for measurement of aripiprazole was shown to be accurate and sensitive. The peaks of aripiprazole (14.21 min) and IS (4.85 min) were well resolved and there were no interfering peaks at the retention times of IS and analyte in the blank plasma sample (Fig.10.1). Excellent linearity was observed between the peak area ratio and drug concentration over the range 20–400 ng/ml and a linear equation in the form $y = 0.0042x–0.0087$ derived by least square regression analysis (Fig.10.2), where x is the spiked concentration and y is peak area ratio of aripiprazole to Internal Standard.

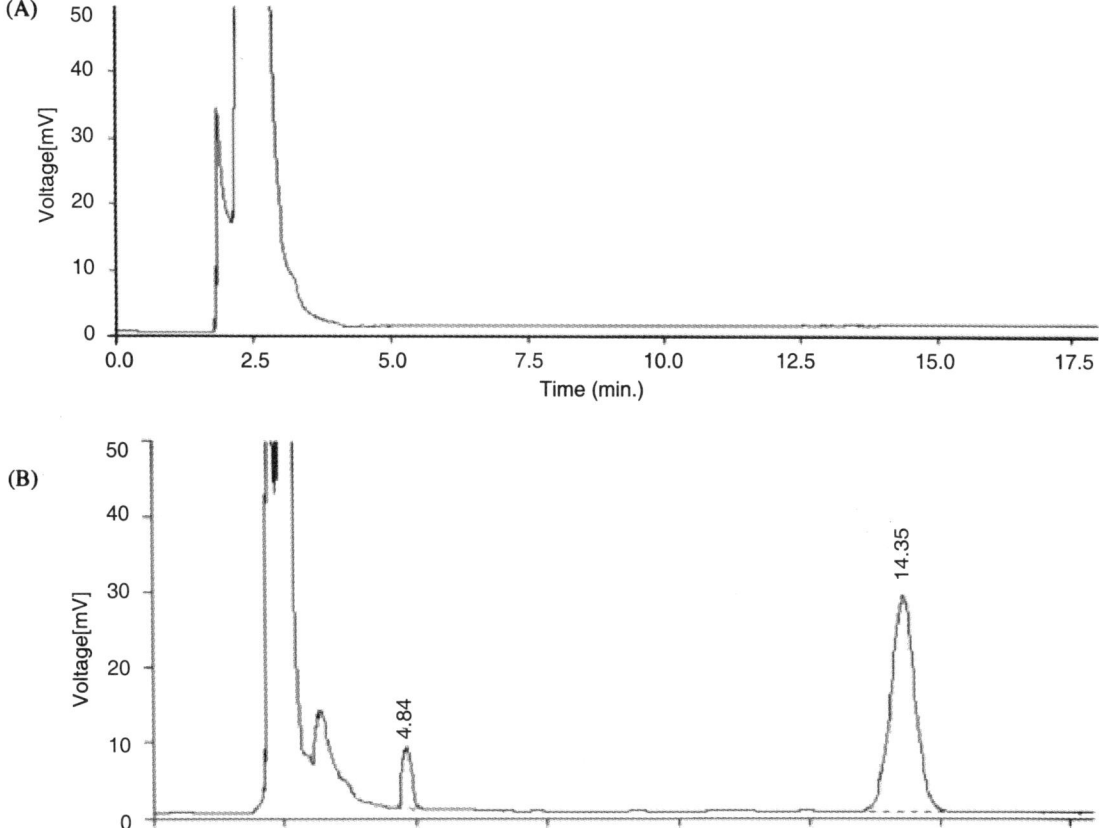

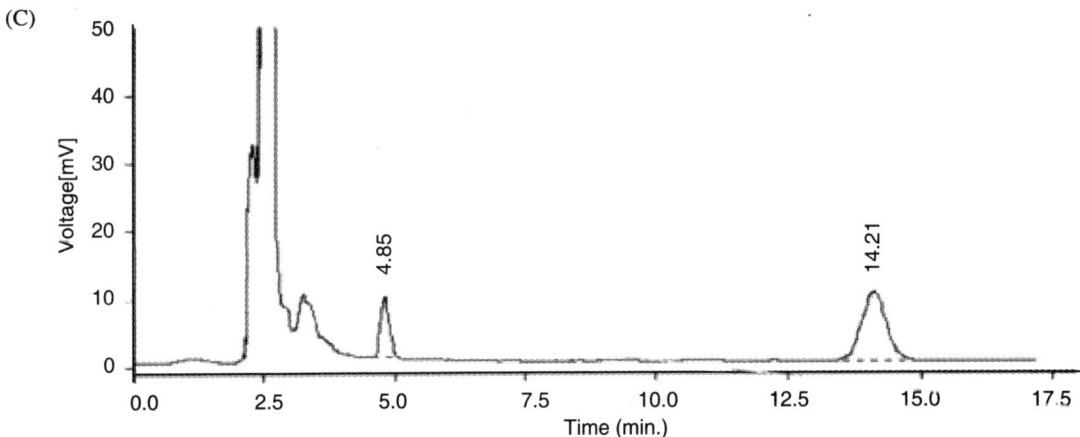

Fig. 10.1. Chromatograms of (A) Blank plasma, (B) Blank plasma spiked with 200 ng/ml of aripiprazole, (C) Volunteer plasma containing 99 ng/ml of aripiprazole after administration of 30 mg aripiprazole tablet. Retention time of IS are at 4.84 (B) and 4.85 (C); Retention time of aripiprazole are at 14.35 (B) and 14.21 (C); No interfering peaks at retention time of IS and aripiprazole in the chromatogram of blank plasma.

The linearity achieved for this assay (20 to 400 ng/ml) effectively covers the therapeutic range. The lower limit of detection defined as three times the base noise was 10 ng/ml for this analytical method and the limit of quantitation was 20 ng/ml (n = 13, SD = 1.09). The sensitivity of the assay was sufficient for determination of aripiprazole in human plasma for a period of 1 to 48 hours.

Between–run and within–run accuracy were over 95% and their % CV did not exceed 10%. Freeze thaw recovery was found to be suitable for this study.

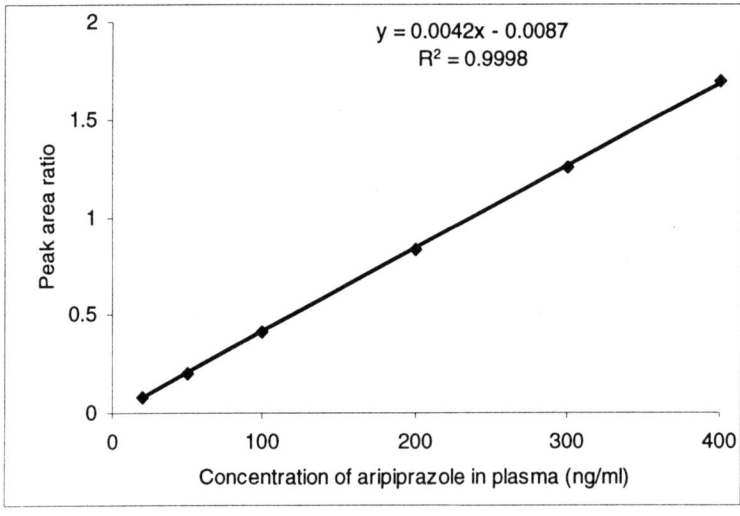

Fig. 10.2. Calibration curve of aripiprazole in plasma

Figure 10.3 shows the mean aripiprazole concentration versus time profile after oral administration of single dose of 30 mg aripiprazole for both brands (standard and test).

The mean pharmacokinetic parameters of all the 12 human volunteers are tabulated in Table 10.6. It is evident from the Table that all the pharmacokinetic parameters (C_{max}, t_{max}, AUC_{0-t}, AUC_{0-t}, K_{el} and $t_{1/2}$) are found to be most comparable with those of reference preparation. The 90% confidence interval (CI) for C_{max}, AUC_{0-t} and AUC_{o-inf} values of test and reference preparation (Table 10.7) were within the accepted limit of DCGI guidelines (0.8–1.2).

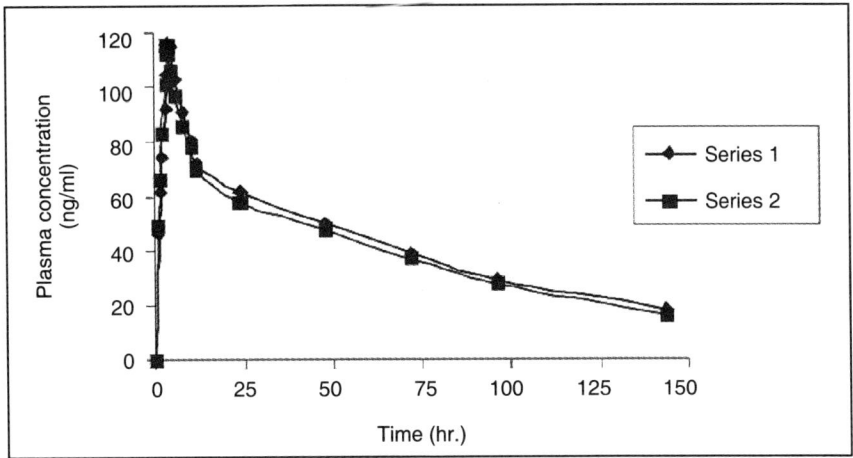

Fig 10.3. Mean plasma concentration *versus* time (hr) of aripiprazole 30 mg tablet (Test and Reference) oral administration to 12 human volunteers for reference and test preparation

Table 10.6: Mean pharmacokinetic parameter obtained in 12 healthy volunteers after the administration of both 30 mg aripiprazole test and reference formulations

Pharmacokinetic Parameter	Reference Preparation (A)		Test Preparation (B)	
$AUC_{0-\infty}$ (ng.hr/ml)	Mean	7249.7455	Mean	7266.750
	± SD	1480.641	± SD	2146.7847
AUC_{0-t} (ng.hr/ml)	Mean	5049.3744	Mean	4962.6749
	± SD	902.5292	± SD	1189.5371
C_{max} (ng/ml)	Mean	119.35	Mean	118.82
	± SD	16.007	± SD	20.764
t_{max} (hr)	Mean	3.8333	Mean	3.9583
	± SD	0.5365	± SD	0.6895
K_{el} (hr^{-1})	Mean	0.0139	Mean	0.013834
	± SD	0.0019	± SD	0.00247
$t_{1/2}$ (hr)	Mean	50.5778	Mean	51.6874
	± SD	7.949	± SD	9.804
Relative bioavailability (%)	100		98.28	

Table 10.7: The 90% confidence interval of various pharmacokinetic parameters of test and reference formulation of aripiprazole 30 mg tablet

C_{max}	Untransformed Data	0.87–1.09
	Ln transformed Data	0.97–1.02
AUC_{0-t}	Untransformed Data	0.85–1.11
	Ln transformed Data	0.98–1.01
$AUC_{0-\infty}$	Untransformed Data	0.86–1.14
	Ln transformed Data	0.98–1.01

On the basis of comparison of AUC_{0-t} for aripiprazole 30 mg after single dose administration, the relative bioavailability of test preparation of tablet aripiprazole 30 mg was 98.282965% to that of reference preparation and the test preparation was bioequivalent to reference preparation.

During the whole study, no serious adverse effects were observed; although postural dizziness and blood pressure lowering have been observed in some of the volunteers (2 out of 12 volunteers) but ECG reports confirm the non-significant physiological change. Moreover, it is not also statistically significant.

ACKNOWLEDGEMENT

The authors are thankful to Psycho Remedies, Ludhiana, India for offering the job of bioequivalence study by supplying test sample and Ranbaxy Solus, New Delhi, India for supplying their brand product. The DCGI is also thanked for the approval of this study.

REFERENCES

1. U.S. Department of Health and Human Services, Food and Drug Administration Center for Veterinary Medicine (CVM), October 10, 2000.

2. U.S. Department of Health and Human Services, Food and Drug Administration Center for Veterinary Medicine (CVM), October 10, 2000.

3. Food and Drug Administration of the United States, *Guidance for industry-Bioanalytical Method Validation*, U.S. Department of Health and Human Services, Center for Drug Evaluation and Research (CDER), Center for Veterinary Medicine (CVM), May 2001 (htpp://www.fda.gov/cder/guidance/index.htm).

4. International conference of harmonization; htpp//www.ich.org.

5. Burris K.D., Molski T.F., Xu C., Ryan E., Tottori K., Kikuchi T., Aripiprazole, a novel antipsychotic, is a high affinity partial agonist at human dopamine D2 receptors. J Pharmacol Exp Ther. 302: 381-389, 2002.

6. Jordan S., Koprivica V., Chen R., Tottori K., Kikuchi T., Altar C.A., The antipsychotic aripiprazole is a potent, partial agonist at the human 5-HT$_{1A}$ receptors. Eur J Pharmacol. 441: 137-140, 2002.

7. McQuade R., Burris K.D., Jordan S., Tottori K., Kurahashi N., Kikuchi T., Aripiprazole: a dopamine-serotonin system stabilizer.Int j Neuropsychopharm. 5 (suppl. 1): S176, 2002.

8. Lawler C.P., Prioleau C., Lewis M.M., Mak C., Jiang D., Schetz J.A., Interactions of the novel antipsychotic aripiprazole (OPC-14597) with dopamine and serotonin receptors subtypes. Neuropsychopharmacology. 20: 612-627, 1999.

9. Citrome L, Josiassen R., Bark N., et al., Pharmacokinetics and safety of aripiprazole and concomitant mood stabilizers. International Journal of Neuropsychopharmacology. 5 (Suppl. 1): S187, 2002 Jun.

10. Mallikaarjun S., Salazar D.E., Bramer S.L., Pharmacokinetics, tolerability, and safety of aripiprazole following single and multiple oral dose administration. European Neuropsychopharmacology. 10 (Suppl. 3): 306-7, 2000 Sept.

11. Mallikaarjun S., Ali M.W., Salazar D.E., et al., The effects of age and gender on the pharmacokinetics of aripiprazole. Clin Pharmacol Ther. 71(2):66, 2002 Feb.

12. Auby P., Saha A.R., Mirza A., et al., Safety and tolerability of aripiprazole at doses higher than 30 mg. Eur. Neuropsychopharmacol. 12 (Suppl. 3):S288, 2002.

13. Daniel D.G., Saha A.R., Ingenito G., et al., Aripiprazole, a novel antipsychotic: overview of a phase II study result. International Journal of Neuropsychopharmacology. 3 (Suppl. 1): S157, 2000 July.

14. Mallikaarjun S., Daniel E.S., Steven L.B., Pharmacokinetics, Tolerability, and Safety of Aripiprazole following Multiple Oral Dosing in Normal Healthy Volunteers. Journal of Clinical Pharmacology. 44: 179-187, 2004.

15. Pal T.K., Mandal U., Ganesan M., Jaykumar M., Chattaraj T.K., Roy K., Banerjee S., Bioequivalence Study of Rabeprazole Sodium on Healthy Human Volunteers. Journal of The Indian Medical Association. 102(1): 26-30, 2003 Jan.

16. Pal T.K., Mandal U., Ganesan M., Jaykumar M., Chattaraj T.K., Roy K., Banerjee S., High performance liquid chromatographic determination of COX-2 inhibitor Rafecoxib in Human plasma. Journal of The Indian Medical Association. 101(08): 486-88, 2003 March.

17. Pal T.K., Mandal U., Musmade P., Ghosh A., Chakraborty Mita., Senthil Rajan D., Jaykumar M., Chakraborty M., Chattaraj T. K., Roy K., Banerjee S., A Study to Determine the Pharmacokinetics of Gatifloxacin following a single oral Dose. Journal of The Indian Medical Association. 102: 488-490, 2004 Sept.

Chapter 11

Drug Information and Clinical Research

Krishnangshu Ray

1

A path-breaking bill seeking to provide right to information was passed by the Lok Sabha on Wednesday, May 11, 2005. Any medicine is a chemical entity with some information hidden in it. Rational and judicious uses of medicines and their rightful consumption are possible, provided the prescriber, dispenser or consumer is well informed. In spite of limited lists of 354 essential medicines, Indian drug market is flooded with 60,000 formulations which in comparison has been restricted to only three to four thousands in most of the Western countries. Out of this vast sellable number of drugs in India only 5% are considered truly useful, 10% are sophisticated costly remedies and the majority of the rest are considered non-effective, unscientific or even harmful. In a developing country like us drug is probably a minor index of priority while compared to literacy, nutritional status, safe drinking water or environmental sanitation. Considering the poor accessibility of information resources on these plethora of medicines, the role of Drug Information Services could be of paramount importance.

What?

'Drug Information' is defined as an objective, scientifically derived and documented data of knowledge involving the pharmacological, toxicological and therapeutic consumption of drugs. It comprises information such as chemical name, structure, identification, dynamic and kinetic properties, indication, interaction, dosage schedule, comparative and clinical data pertinent to the diagnosis and treatment of patients. Drug Information Services (DIS) include the gathering, reviewing, evaluating, indexing, organizing, summarizing and distributing information on drugs in various forms by various methods to its actual and potential users.

When?

The first official Drug Information Center (DIC) was established in North America in 1962. Subsequently, several health professionals in the field of Medicine and Pharmacy jointly contemplated to organize such centers in major hospitals of USA. Clinical pharmacists of the hospitals were chosen to act as the leaders of such program including the development of patient profiles, unit-dose drug distribution system and liaison between the prescribers and the nurses. WHO in its meeting in 1991 at

Madrid resolved to form an International Society of Drug Bulletins (ISDB) amongst its member states for networking between the independent drug bulletins disseminating drug information. In India there exist not more than 20 such centers of which Govt. sponsored Centers are handful. DIDC, Kolkata is first of its kind in Eastern region which is totally supported by the Sector Investment Project, Dept. of Health.

Why?

DIDC functions as the communication network to bridge between the wealth of current information available and the health professional acting as end-users. It facilitates the prescribers to access the data in a highly specific and efficient manner to enable them in arriving at a quicker and more rational decisions. Drug Information Services could be of active or passive varieties. Active dissemination occurs when relevant information is passed on directly to the physicians usually at the bed-side to facilitate immediate patient-care interaction. Passive dissemination is considered as pharmacist responding to the queries received at the center. The organization and the content of the center would depend upon the category of the user, e.g. whether it is patient-oriented, clinician-oriented or community-oriented. A community DIC acts as a resource base for the questions on poisoning, drug abuse, OTC products, rational administration of medications and adverse effects.

How?

Organizationally, a simple DIC could be equipped with a few desks, shelves, filing cabinets, a telephone, a computer with an internet connection and a photocopier. Access to a medical library and essential telephone numbers such as Poison Control Centers, referral hospitals with telemedicine facilities are also desirable. Regarding the human resources for an ideal DIC at least one trained pharmacist must be employed to operate the center. The person should have sound pharmaceutical knowledge base blended with clinical aptitudes, familiarity to information technology and excellent communication skill. The expertise is usually developed through the combination of formal training and hand-on education. This determines the number and type of questions and also identifies the major users of this service. The reference sources of the DIC may be Tertiary (Textbooks, Pharmacopoea, Formularies), Secondary (Abstracts) or Primary (Journals, Research Papers). Besides the print media both on-line computer softwares like Med-line, Drug-line, Drug-dex, Tox-line, etc. or CD-ROM systems must be installed. Other comprehensive modalities like Iowa Drug Information Services (IDIS) or Paul deHaen Drug Information Service, etc. could be other retrieval services.

DIDC: Outputs?

DIDC, Kolkata has emerged as a Government referral unit for every stakeholders related to drug uses. Principally all services provided by DIDC are free of users charges. Instead of serving queries other outputs are:

   (*i*) Publication of Bengali handbook "Oshudh Niye" for lay consumers which compiled every aspects of drug consumption, sale, legal importance and problem-based therapeutics

  (*ii*) Publication of English Newsletter "Infomedex" for all categories of health professionals (doctors, nurses, pharmacists) working at the primary health care levels. The issues incorporates pertinent ailments of primary care and their management

 (*iii*) Preparation of "Hospital Formulary" of Government catalogue drugs

 (*iv*) Conducting epidemiological researches or KAP study (Knowledge, Attitude and Practice) of drug consumption by consumers (*v*) Study of Drug Utilization Patterns in hospital practices

(*vi*) Contributing in the framing of State Drug Policy Draft, Standard Treatment Protocols (STP) for primary care diseases

(*vii*) Acting as a tool in the field of Medical Education by optimum utilization by under and post-graduate students

Prospects

The center may be responsible for organizing Journal Clubs, Educational CMEs periodically to keep all concerned up-to-date about new drug developments. This can be accomplished by publication of Newsletters, Bulletins, etc. Drug utilization data from various hospitals and community could identify the apparent under or overuse of particular drugs. Comparative data from different region or country expressed by anatomical therapeutic chemical (ATC) classification or internationally defined daily doses (DDD) furnishes patterns of prescribing. Drug utilization data and Market Research Statistics that are available at DIC can also be valuable indicators of the effectiveness of activities to educate and inform prescribers (Feedback study) through the articles in the bulletins.

SUMMARY

The cardinal objectives of DIC are to develop and disseminate unbiased, truthful and scientific information about rational drugs to all stakeholders like Drug Industry, Govt. Regulatory Agency, the Medical Community, Drug Retailers and other Consumer Groups. To achieve the aforesaid objectives both the Industry and the Government must provide complete information about all registered drugs including their consumption patterns (Drug Utilization Data). WHO recommends that an ideal DIC should be established in a teaching hospital which is resourced by library back-up, Academia and Information Technology facilities like Broad banding and Telemedicine. The role of independent print media like independent drug bulletins published by the DIC should also be acknowledged. Collaboration with the Government eventually plays a vital role in formulating the Rational Drug and Health Policy. The organizers of such centers are expected to generate awareness amongst both actual and potential users of it. The success indictors of any DIC depends upon gradual increase in the number of its users in one hand and the conversion of potential users to actual users on the other.

Clinical Research with Drugs: Prospects and Perspective

<table>
<tr><td>2</td><td style="text-align:right">Parthasarathi Bhattacharyya</td></tr>
</table>

I was a little surprised at the invitation for this write up. Clinical research, itself is a sort of speciality and I am hardly better than a novice to deal with this subject. Hence, I felt comfortable to write from the perspective of a practising physician.

To a physician clinical research means either dealing with a disease or doing some clinical trial with drugs. By virtue of a little interest in drug trial he may know the four phases of it. He can, perhaps, make out the areas of concern as to find out safety, efficacy, adverse effects, dose, indications, contraindication, drug-drug interaction, etc. – involved in a drug trial. By performing a phase III or IV trial, he may have experienced the need for being meticulous in documentation and need of communication with the CRO, etc. Some of the interested and able physicians may carry out phase III and IV trials in our country, a few may have done phase II even but for a practising doctor, I do not think that doing phase I trial is possible.

The scientific aptitude of a physician can carry him with innovative ideas to play with drugs ethically in certain circumstances. He or she can try an empirical treatment at certain situations and make record of the patients to end up in a personal experience file. Treating fever with skin rash as mycoplasma infection was one such good experience of mine in a district hospital. In early ninetees there was a breakout of enteric fever and we treated them with ciprofloxacin successfuly though nobody tought us to do so. The maximum available investigation was Widal test which does not come positive before the second week of the disease. Observation of relapse of fever in such patients leads us to treat them with antitubercular drugs and we proved our stand correct on prospective documentation of Mantoux conversion. Well, these records are silently forgotten though the community benefitted tremendously in crisis. At the end of the story, the unregulated prescription market could make cipro-resistant enteric emerge quickly and no clinical research looked into the mode of development and steps of prevention of such a wrong thing. We must know that the priority to a clinician should be the right way of use of drug and not in performing a drug trial or using a drug in an innovative way. Ironically, this important applied aspect of operational research is neglected. A physician in India can try methetroxate in Indian sarcoidosis patients as a replication of its use in USA or Europe. Thus, he does a clinical research unaware and gets recognition once he or she can publish it after proper documentation. Some doctor from a South Indian Institute made news and controversy by using sildenafil in babies with pulmonary hypertension. Sildenafil is now recognized as a treatment of pulmonary hypertension from several causes. Thanks to the innovative use — a wonderful piece of clinical research: the scientific basis was strong, the use was ethical and the motive was humane.

As for myself in my institute we do a lot of practice of clinical science. Operational research is simple – like questionnaire based studies. Despite limitations, audit of the compliance to therapy for any chronic ailment (e.g. asthma) is of immense importance. Similarly, we enjoyed the job of developing endobronchial sealing — a new mode of treating hemoplysis. We also described a higher prevalence of relaxation abnormality of left ventricle (diastolic dysfunction) in advanced COPD patients who benefit from a drug called diltiazem.

Well, beyond all these, a physician can opt to be a co-ordinator or a principal investigator (PI) in a trial whatever be the phase. The role as a PI is not easy. It involves a lot of responsibilities and commitments often not adequately compensated by the so called financial or other advantage. The job of a PI starts from making a proposal and negotiation with a CRO, knowing regulatory requirements and the facts of compliance assessments too. He is a key contributor to the protocol preparation, review and approval.

He is the person for training of the working staff, patient recruitment and registration. Apart he has the sole responsibility for conducting the protocol, taking care of the ancillary services, billing, budget management, reporting the results, arranging equipment supply/procurement, administration, account establishment and close out with all financial appraisals. Finally the PI has to get into the manuscript preparation and publication. In a nutshell, the grass is not all green; it is green; only once you are capable and ready to afford time and inputs. To me, drug trials are to be dealt with people who are sincere and serious about it.

It all sounds nice when someone boasts of his or her involvement and success in drug trials. They are easy in one way since the CROs involved take up a lot of their problems. But, in a drug trial, a physician is like a caged tiger. He is bound by the protocol and he has no choice to go beyond that to cherish his own options or innovations. There is no dearth of such physicians who cherish to get involved in different clinical, epidemiological and operational research beyond drug trials. I find the following problems for them:

1. Lack of knowledge of finding authorities
2. Lack of legal knowledge
3. Lack of statistical support
4. Lack of access to appropriate manpower
5. Lack of access to literature
6. Lack of environment and research culture
7. Lack of locally available defined guidelines
8. Lack of time

All these lacunae are the hindrances of clinical research development and prosperity in our country. When I look as a physician to solve them, I appreciate that the following could be done as a priority:

I. **Grooming:** Let there be a defined approach in medical schools. Let this issue be incorporated at least as a chapter in medicine and/or pharmacology. Let there be a small operational desertation for all MBBS candidates.

II. **Establishment of a core help station in each state:** This will provide all possible logistic and intellectual support to the researchers.

III. **Establishment of a central independent ethics committee in each state:** This will deal with all protocols quickly. It may be partly state sponsored to encourage clinical research. Some lavy may be charged by the state for CRO sponsored drug trials for ethical clearance, review, monitoring, etc.

IV. Establishment of a central review committee of the state.

V. Involvement of industries and universities in the process.

VI. Encouraging innovative research in biomedical instrumentation, etc.

VII. Ayurvedic research.

VIII. Finally set all the grants visible from a single window. Anybody can log on to the resources at any point of time.

Today, a physician is at the crossroads of clinical research. In one hand drug trials are going to pour in through which we can improve national economy. Simultaneously by performing other aspects of clinical research, we can usher a new era of improved treatment of ailments and preserve national health.

The government, the policy makers, and the intelligentsia should act fast and firm. We have unlimited human resource to get to the top of the world.

Overview of the Drug Discovery and Development Process

<table>
<tr><td>3</td><td>Avijit Hazra</td></tr>
</table>

ABSTRACT

In the modern world, drug discovery and development is a multidisciplinary, creative, complex and highly-regulated process. Although much of the new drug development is being undertaken by the research-based pharmaceutical industry, the basic research driving generation of leads is still undertaken in research laboratories and academic institutions. Once a lead has been generated, it is optimized and the new molecular entities subjected to a battery of routine and special toxicity tests in animals. The technical and moral reservations against intact animal testing is increasingly prompting use of alternatives such as cell and tissue culture testing and *in silico* modeling using advanced computer simulations. Nevertheless the need for animal testing is likely to continue into the foreseeable future. When a drug candidate has successfully cleared animal tests, it begins a series of stepwise clinical trials in healthy human volunteers and patients. If the safety and effectiveness can be established in comparison to placebo or standard treatment, marketing authorization is granted by the regulatory agency at the end of phase III trials. However, postmarketing surveillance continues, sometimes as formal clinical trials but more often as passive surveillance, throughout the lifetime of the product as a marketed medicine. The huge attrition rates between the library of molecular leads and the medicine on the chemist's shelves means that the drug development process is complex, time-consuming and expensive. The rewards are correspondingly high if an unmet therapeutic need can be genuinely fulfilled. The Indian academia and pharmaceutical industry must gear up and join hands to face the challenge of new drug development, backed by a supportive regulatory environment.

INTRODUCTION

In the modern world, drug discovery and development is a creative, complex and highly regulated process. On average, it can take upwards of 10 years to navigate a medication from the laboratory to the chemist's shelves. Although the development of new technologies has provided opportunities to significantly shorten that timeline, the process remains scientifically complex and elaborate.

Although most new drug development today is being undertaken by the pharmaceutical industry, much of the basic work for understanding the pathophysiology of disease and identifying possible disease targets for attenuation by drugs is carried on in universities, academic institutions and public sector research laboratories.

Participants in the New Drug Development Process

New drug development is one of the most intense multidisciplinary scientific activities that is undertaken by man. Chemists, botanists, microbiologists, information technology professionals, pharmaceutical scientists and engineers, pharmacologists, toxicologists, clinicians (doctors), legal experts, regulatory affair experts, financial managers, are all involved in the process. Clinical pharmacologists serve as the link while transferring the drug from the laboratory to the bedside.

Generating Leads

This refers to the process of designing and synthesizing novel compounds based on desired properties. Traditionally, it begins in a researcher's laboratory, through selection and examination of specific biological targets. These targets are disease-relevant, which means they play an important role in the progression of a disease or its symptoms. Researchers try to design or find molecules that act on the target, which then undergo extensive laboratory testing to determine their activity on the target. Those who interact desirably become potential candidates for further study. Multiple compounds are usually identified and tested to determine which have the desired profile. Lead candidates are those with promising characteristics that 'lead the way' to develop new drugs.

In the past, researchers were limited by the number of leads they had access to and the speed with which these could be assessed. With the advent of high-throughput technologies, the number of compounds and speed of assessment has increased significantly.

Optimizing Leads

'Optimizing' the lead refers to the process used to manipulate the compound to improve its biological or therapeutic properties. The chemical structure is modified to generate molecules that can be produced as the dosage forms for use in preclinical studies, which confirm the compound's biological activity, safety, toxicology and pharmacokinetic profile. The process of 'optimizing' leads concludes with the selection of an Early Development Candidate (EDC), which is the drug candidate selected for more intense study, beginning with animals.

Toxicity Testing and Animal Studies

The purpose of toxicity testing of drugs is to ensure that a product is safe when used as directed. The results of these tests also provide scientific data for poison control centers and emergency room personnel should a product be misused.

Toxicology is the study of the harmful effects of substances on living systems. Toxicologists test prescription drugs, over-the-counter drugs, food additives, household products, pesticides, chemicals and cosmetics, including cosmeceuticals like sunscreen, antiperspirants and dandruff shampoo. The relative safety of a substance is judged according to its effects under different variations of dose, route of administration, duration and frequency of exposure.

The question whether we really need to use animals for testing is hotly debated. Because scientists have drastically reduced the number of animals needed for product safety testing, animal rights activists have led the public to believe that the use of laboratory animals can be eliminated from this field altogether. This is far from the truth at the moment. It is often important to understand how the living system as a whole responds to drugs, including how repair and defense mechanisms operate in case the drug is causing toxicity. Therefore, promising drug candidates are put through a battery of animal toxicity tests and also assessed for effectiveness in suitable animal models of disease.

In vitro testing and some alternatives to the use of animals have proven to be of value in this work, but the fact remains that most such alternatives can only be used to screen for selected toxic effects. In the final analysis, some animal models must be used to assess the drug's effectiveness and suitability for testing in man. While scientific societies have issued strong statements in support of the development of non-animal methodologies, they also caution that there are no known validated alternatives to the use of animals for the assessment of lethal potency and acute toxicity. Nor are such alternatives likely to appear in the near future. Therefore, not performing adequate intact animal testing places people as well as animals at risk.

Types of toxicity tests

The nature and extent of testing of a new chemical entity (NCE) may vary from one type of product to another. The intended use of the product, the ways in which humans are likely to be exposed to it, the specific properties of the product and the dictates of laws and regulations are all factors in determining which tests are needed and the extent of product safety evaluation.

Further, because of the risk of accidental overexposure or poisoning, toxicologists need to know how a substance affects the body in overdose. Careful observation of the experimental animals and analysis of body chemistry provides this essential information. Subsequent autopsy provides data on toxicity to various organ systems.

The usual toxicity tests are **acute toxicity**, including assessment of lethality, **skin and eye irritancy (Draize) tests** and **subacute** and **chronic toxicity** studies that examine the risks of extended exposure to new chemicals and drugs. **Teratology** and **reproductive toxicity** studies assess a chemical's potential to cause birth defects. **Mutagenicity** and **genotoxicity** studies assess the tendency to cause adverse changes in the genetic makeup of an organism. **Carcinogenicity** studies evaluate the cancer-causing risk on extended exposure.

The LD_{50} test: The median lethal dose (LD_{50}) test is a measure of acute lethality–how much of the substance and under what conditions it can cause immediate illness, injury and death. An LD_{50} rating is calculated for the dose at which one half of the test animals can be expected to die following the ingestion of the test substance.

The use of the "classic" LD_{50} test, developed more than fifty years ago, although statistically more precise, is now discouraged. The "limit" test which uses 10 to 20 animals, not 80 to 100 animals like the "classic" LD_{50}, has become the standard. In this test, animals are given a single dose or, if necessary, a few equally spaced doses of the chemical within a 24-hour period. The dose given relates to body weight. The majority of test animals are rodents (mice and rats). Although the results of the "limit" test may not be as precise, this form of testing is usually a sufficient replacement for the "classic" LD_{50}.

Non-animal Alternatives for Product Safety Testing

For economic and ethical reasons, there is active commitment to refine existing tests to minimize animal distress, reduce animal usage, replace whole-animal testing and to search for more of these alternatives. Before any non-animal method can be accepted as an "alternative", its value as a genuine substitute has to be validated. The pharmaceutical industry actively supports efforts to develop and evaluate promising non-animal procedures. The scientific community has been successful in reducing the number of animals used in safety testing as well as in refining test methods to reduce any pain or distress these animals may experience. However, each alternative method has its limitations.

Mathematical models can help to predict an organism's responses to varying levels of exposure to a particular substance. They can also help in improving the design of scientific experiments. These models are no substitute for observation of the effects of a substance in a complex living system.

Computer data banks allow for the reduction of test duplication. They are also useful in the initial evaluation of chemicals slated for further study; unsuitable chemicals can be eliminated from consideration prior to the institution of animal testing. Unfortunately, computers can only process and store existing knowledge – much of which come from animal studies. Animal testing is needed to expand that knowledge base.

Cells, tissues and even whole organs obtained from animals and humans can be used for preliminary screening of chemical compounds. They can help identify substances that are so toxic that there is no purpose in continuing to investigate them. *In vitro* tests cannot reveal the effects of a substance on a complex living organism composed of many different organs and systems. In the end, the validity of such tests must be verified by testing on an appropriate intact, living organism.

Microorganisms and lower invertebrates—single-cell organisms such as protozoa and bacteria are increasingly useful in early screening for toxic effects. Because of their simple physiology, they shed little light on complex toxicity questions, and thus are less useful in late stages of testing protocols. Invertebrate animals such as insects and mollusks are also useful in preliminary tests, but the results obtained are often too general to be applied to multiorgan toxicity problems in humans.

Clinical Trials

Once a NCE satisfactorily completes the essential toxicity and other preclinical tests, it becomes an investigational new drug (IND) that is now to be investigated in man through the process of clinical trials. Clinical testing is highly regulated by government agencies and codes for the conduct of clinical trials are specifically outlined in official documents, e.g. Schedule Y of the Indian Drugs & Cosmetics Act of 1940, as amended from time to time. Trial protocols have to be designed carefully and necessary ethical clearances sought before human experimentation can beginning. Simultaneously with clinical testing, concurrent analytical and technical development is undertaken (see Boxes) to scale up production of the new substance, define analytical methodologies, and take care of other pharmaceutical aspects. In addition, long-term and special toxicity testing may also be undertaken depending upon the intended use.

The clinical trial process is separated into different phases, each with a specific objective. Initial human tests, called phase I studies, usually involve a small number (20 to 50) of healthy volunteers, and are conducted to determine dosing levels and assess the safety, tolerability, dose response and metabolic properties of the compound in humans. This must be undertaken only in an indoor hospital setting with backup of intensive care facilities. If the drug proposed to be tested has a high potential of causing toxicity, such as anticancer drugs, even Phase I studies are to be carried out in patients rather than volunteers.

In phase II studies (therapeutic exploratory trials), the drug is administered to a larger number (50 to 500) of subjects, usually spread over multiple centers. They are intended to confirm the drug's safety profile in patients diagnosed with the disease being studied. Phase II studies can be divided into two categories: smaller phase II studies (sometimes called phase IIa pilot studies) usually examine a variety of doses to identify the initial dosing regimen. Larger phase II studies confirm the safety in a larger patient population, and define the optimum dosing regimen. Because they are often randomized, double blind studies, they also provide preliminary data on the drug's efficacy. The caveat is that the patient population selected for phase II are usually homogenous with a minimum of comorbidities and use of concurrent medication.

Concurrent Technical Development—Analytical Studies

- Analytical method development and validation
- Chromatography (HPLC & GC with various detectors, LC/MS, TLC)
- Spectroscopy (FT-IR, AAS, polarimetry, UV/VIS)
- Drug substance characterization
- Comparator studies

- Stability sample analysis
- Dissolution testing
- Release testing
- Raw material testing
- Identification of impurities and residual solvents
- Elucidation of the degradation pathways
- Methods transfer
- Vitamin and mineral assays
- Total carbon analysis

Phase III studies (therapeutic confirmatory trials) are much larger in scale, and gather additional information about the drug's safety and effectiveness in the intended patient population. Depending on the therapeutic area, a few thousand of patients may be enrolled extending across multiple centers. A limited range of comorbidities and concurrent medication is permitted to mimic real-life situation. The drug being tested is usually compared to placebo or to one or more currently available therapies. The usual design is randomized double-blind study, with the groups being tested in parallel or crossed-over with an adequate washout period in between. The objective is to show statistical superiority, or at least non-inferiority, in efficacy or safety over current or dummy treatments. In addition to assessing effectiveness in closer-to-real life situation, phase III studies usually quantify the incidence of common adverse drug reactions (ADRs) and detect less common ADRs, interaction with common illnesses and interaction with concomitant medication.

This critical endpoints of Phase III studies are needed to obtain regulatory approval to market the drug. In spite of the fact that phase III trials are one of the last important steps before requesting marketing approval, drug candidates may still be discontinued if the study results are negative. Discontinuing drug development at such a late stage in the process contributes to the enormous cost of bringing drugs to market.

Concurrent Technical Development—Preformulation Studies

- Moisture sorption curves
- Solubility profiles
- pKa
- Partition coefficients
- Excipient compatibility studies
- Production scaling studies

Submission and Approval

Data collected from the preclinical and clinical studies are compiled into reports for review and approval by governmental regulatory agencies. These reports, which represent the official request for marketing authorization, comprise the New Drug Application (NDA) in the United States of America and Marketing Authorization Application (MAA) in many other countries. The regulatory agency in a country determines whether the studies conducted and the results obtained support the indication requested. Once the application is approved, the company is allowed to market the drug but only for the specific indication(s) outlined in the package insert. The approval process may take 2 to 3 years unless 'fast-track' reviews are done for particularly important drugs. Additional data, and hence studies, may be required during this phase to satisfy regulatory requirements.

The huge costs of drug development have prompted countries with the major share of the research-based pharmaceutical industry, namely USA, the European Union countries and Japan, to formulate the International Conference on Harmonization (ICH) of regulatory requirements for pharmaceuticals intended for human use. If these common guidelines are followed, duplication of testing can be avoided when the drug is sought to be marketed in different countries. ICH good clinical practice guidelines are now the norms guiding clinical development in the advanced countries.

Further Clinical Trials

Clinical trials do not end once a drug is launched. Phase IIIb studies may be performed after an application for marketing approval has been submitted, but before the approval has been granted. These clinical trials are performed within the proposed indications and dosages, and are not intended for primary registration purposes.

Phase IV studies are conducted following approval to provide additional supporting data to complement the product profile or to extend indications. Thus phase IV trials may be conducted to assess safety and effectiveness in special patient groups like children, elderly, expectant or nursing mothers, who are not involved in initial clinical development; assess long term morbidity-mortality; quality of life assessments; pharmacoeconomic studies and bioequivalence studies. The majority of phase IV studies are, however, in the nature of passive surveillance (postmarketing surveillance) for further qualification of ADRs, detection of rare and delayed ADRs and for assessment of interaction with various illnesses and various drugs.

In essence, once a new drug is approved and launched in the market, it continues to be in surveillance throughout its lifespan as a marketed medicine. There are many instances of a drug being withdrawn after lunch owing to recognition of unacceptable ADRs.

CONCLUSION

A brief overview of the complex process of new drug development in today's world has been given above. It is a multidisciplinary effort with intensive input of intellectual and financial capital. In the Indian context, with the adjustments being imposed by the dictates of the TRIPS era, we must gear up to accept the challenge of new drug development. This is not only to gain a respectable share of the economically rewarding world pharmaceutical market, but also to address our own unmet therapeutic needs in communicable and non-communicable disease segments in a manner that would be acceptable and affordable to our population. Industry academia collaboration for new drug development is the need of the hour today in India.

Chapter 12

Repeated Dose Subchronic Oral Toxicity Study of Aceclofenac Sodium in Experimental Rats (28 days)

S. Darbar, A. Bose, N. Chatterjee, B. Roy,
U. Mandal, T.K. Chattaraj,
T.K. Pal, A. Das

INTRODUCTION

Nonsteroidal anti-inflammatory drugs (NSAIDs) are widely used for the treatment of pain and inflammation. NSAIDs produce their therapeutic effect by inhibiting the cyclooxygenase (COX) enzymes, which are involved in the biosynthesis of prostaglandins (PGs) (Aithal et al[1], 2007; Manov et al[2], 2006; Hussaini et al[3], 2007; Vane[4] 1971; Vane et al[5], 1998). Conventional NSAIDs inhibit both COX-1 and COX-2 at therapeutic doses (Dubols 1998).[6]

Aceclofenac sodium, a prodrug in the aryl-acetic acid class, is a commonly used NSAID in several countries. Aceclofenac is an oral non-steroidal anti-inflammatory drug (NSAID) that is effective in the treatment of painful inflammatory diseases and has been used to treat more than 75 million people worldwide (Brogden et al[7], 1996). Chronic use of aceclofenac, damages gastrointestinal mucosa by irritant action, causing alteration in mucosal permeability and/or suppression of prostaglandin synthesis. Aceclofenac is highly protein and has antipyretic, analgesic, and anti-inflammatory effects, is an inhibitor of arachidonic acid level. The use of oral nonsteroidal anti-inflammatory drugs is associated with upper gastrointestinal complications, particularly perforated and bleeding peptic ulcer (Hawkey[8] 1990). The exact mechanism is not known but it is probably related to the decrease in the fatty acid entering the cell or releasing from the cell.

The present study aimed to evaluate the safety and efficacy of aceclofenac in rats by determining both oral acute and oral subchronic toxicities.

MATERIALS AND METHOD

Drugs and Chemicals

Aceclofenac was obtained from Dey's Medical Stores (Mfg) Ltd, 62, Bondel Road, Kolkata-19, India, Serum levels of Glutamate Pyruvate Transaminase [SGPT], Glutamate Oxaloacetate Transanimase

[SGOT], blood glucose, BUN, were determined by Spectrophotometric Methods. These kits were obtained from Ranbaxy Diagnostic Laboratory Ltd., 86-HPSIDC, Baddi, HP-173205, India.

Experimental Animal

Forty-eight wistar albino rat, i.e. 24 male and 24 female healthy rats weighing 130–150 gms were purchased from Indian Institute of Chemical Biology IICB, Kolkata. The rats were divided into eight groups of 6 rats per sex ($n = 6$) administered the dose of 0 (control), 25, 50 and 100 mg/kg/day for 28 days in each groups. Animals were allowed acclimatization period of 7 days to laboratory conditions prior to the initiation of dosing. Rats were assigned to six per cage sex wise and the individual animal was fur marked with picric acid. The females were nulliparous and not pregnant. The room temperature was maintained at 27±2 °C, 55% humidity, and a 12:12 h light and dark cycle. They were fed with standard laboratory chow (Hindustan Lever Food, Bangalore, India) and provided with water *ad libitum*. The experimental procedures were carried out in strict compliances with the Institutional Animal Ethics Committee's (IAEC) rules and regulation of this institute.

Experimental Design

The rats were divided into the following groups with each containing 6 rats ($n = 6$, both sex each):

Group I Control rats which were fed normal diet and water.
Group II Aceclofenac treated rats (low): 25 mg Aceclofenac/kg/day for 4 weeks.
Group III Aceclofenac treated rats (intermediate): 50 mg Aceclofenac/kg/day for 4 weeks.
Group IV Aceclofenac treated rats (high): 100 mg Aceclofenac/kg/day for 4 weeks.

Acute Toxicity Study

The acute oral toxicity was evaluated following the World Health Organization (WHO) guideline (WHO, 2000) and the Organization of Economic Cooperation and Development (OECD) guideline for chemical testing (OECD, 2001). Briefly, rats were divided into two group of twelve animals six males, six females). The treated group was orally given aceclofenac in a single dose of 2000 mg/kg body weight, while the control group received only water vehicle. The animals were monitored for apparent signs of toxicity for 14 days. The animals that died within this period subjected necrosis. All rats were weighted and sacrificed on the 15th day after administration, and then the vital organs including heart, lungs, liver, kidneys, spleen, adrenals, stomach and sex organs were grossly studies and histopathological examined.

Sub-chronic Toxicity Study

The method was performed following the WHO guideline (WHO, 2000) and the OECD guideline (OECD, 1981). Briefly, male and female rats were randomly divided into four groups of six. The treated group of each sex (males and females) was orally given aceclofenac at the dose of 25, 50, 100 mg/kg body weight daily for 28 days, while control group received the vehicle at the same volume. All rats were observed for apparent signs of toxicity or behavioral alterations during the experiment.

Weekly Body Weight

The body weight of each rat was assessed using a sensitive balance during the acclimatization period, once before commencement of dosing, once weekly during the dosing period and once on the day of sacrifice.

Mortality and Clinical Signs

During the four-week dosing period, all the animals were observed daily for clinical signs and mortality patterns once before dosing, immediately after dosing and up to 4 h after dosing.

Relative Organ Weight

On day 28 the dosing period, all the animals were euthanised by exsanguinations under chloroform anesthesia. Different organs namely the heart, lungs, liver, stomach, kidneys, adrenals, testis and ovary were carefully dissected out and weight in grams (absolute organ weight). Relative organ weight of each animal was then calculated as follows:

$$\text{Relative Organ Weight} = \frac{\text{Absolute organ weight (g)}}{\text{Body weight of rat on sacrifice day (g)}} \times 100$$

Biochemical Analysis

Serum levels of Glutamate Pyruvate Transaminase [SGPT], Glutamate Oxaloacetate Transanimase [SGOT] (Retiman et al[9], 1957), Alkaline Phosphate (ALP) (King[10], 1965), Blood Urea Nitrogen (BUN) (Malloy et al[11], 1937), and blood glucose were determined by using standard analytical kit obtained from Ranbaxy Diagnostic Laboratory Ltd., 86-HPSIDC, Baddi, HP-173205, India.

Haematology

Haematological investigations were carried out prior to sacrifice on completion of dosing period of 28 days from each animal fasted overnight. Blood sample was collected from ratinal orbital sinus following morning using heparin as anticoagulant. Blood sample, thus, obtained was placed on ice followed by centrifugation (4000 rpm) and the plasma fraction was collected for haematological analysis using Serono 9110 automated hematology analyzer (Serono-Baker Diagonstics Inc, Allentown, PA). Blood parameters were quantitated for: (1) Haematologic Factors [Haemoglobin concentration (Hb)], Total Erythrocyte Count (RBC), Total and Differential Leucocyte Count, Reticulocyte Concentration (Rt), Haematocrit (HCT), Mean Corpuscular Volume (MCV), and Mean Corpuscular Hemoglobin (MCH)) (Tables 12.3 and 12.4).

Estimation of Total Protein

Protein estimation was done as per the method of Lowry et al[12], 1951.

Histopathological Analysis

Portions of the liver and kidney were then fixed in buffered form formalin solution, processed through graded alcohol and xylene, and embedded in paraffin wax following the standard microtechnique (Galighar & Kozloff[13], 1971). 5-6 μ sections were made at multiple levels and stained routinely with hematoxylin and eosin. Mounted slides were examined and photographs were taken under a light microscope (Tables 12.1 and 12.2).

Statistical Analysis

The results were expressed as means ± standard deviation (s.d.) and values were calculated for each group and a two-way analysis of variance (ANOVA) was done for each quantitative parameter to determine the significance of inter-group differences (Armitage, P. et al[14], 1985).

RESULTS

Histopathological Analysis

Group I (control)

The normal lobular architectural pattern of the liver section is as shown in Fig. 12.1. The lobulation is modest as a result of the low content of interstitial tissues, and can be determined only with reference to the central vein. Sinusoids at the periphery or the lobule are fused into a reticulum. The hepatocytes are arranged in a series of branching and anastomising perforated laminae to form a labyrinth, between which were sinusoidal spaces. The cytoplasm of the hepatocytes was clearly eosinophilic, with prominent nuclei.

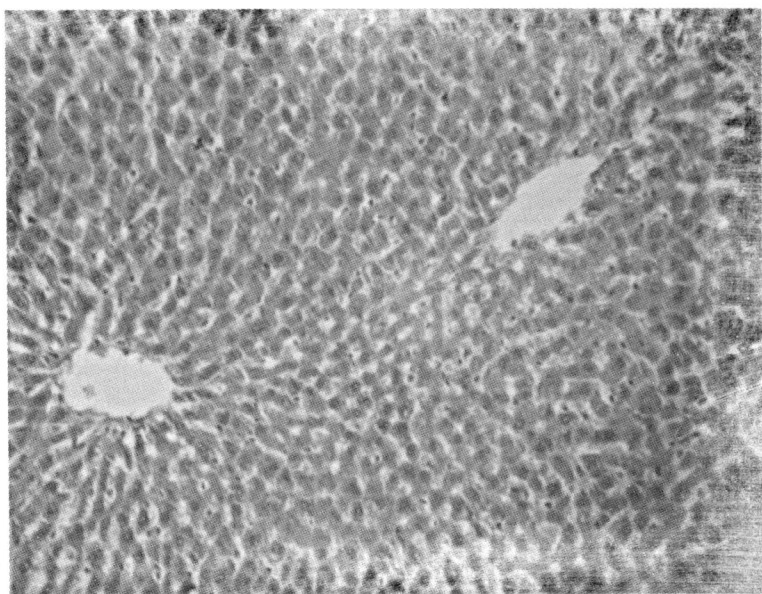

Fig. 12.1. Control rat: LM section of liver showing the normal lobular histological picture (H & E ×100)

Group II (low)

The photomicrograph of the liver section showed a histological picture that closely approximates that of the control group. The plate-like arrangements of the hepatocytes were seen, the sinusoidal spaces were also visible, but not as prominent as in the control group. The cytoplasm of the hepatocyte was clearly eosinophilic as in the control group (Fig. 12.2).

Group III (intermediate)

Mild diarrhoea in the intermediate dose group after 20th day of administration of aceclofenac. Histopathology of rats from intermediate dose group showed similar lesions in liver and kidney but in lesser intensity, i.e., microscopically liver showed loss of normal architecture with vacuolar degeneration of hepatocytes (Fig. 12.3) and the microscopic lesion in kidney was cystic dilatation of collecting tubules with mild vacuolar degeneration of tubular epithelial cells of renal tubules in some of the areas.

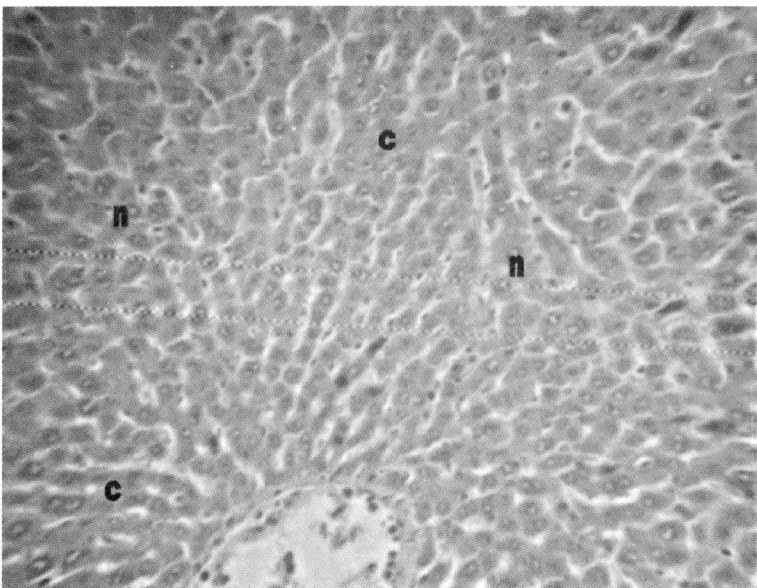

Fig. 12.2. Aceclofenac treated rat (low dose): LM section of liver showing a normal histological picture. Normal hepatocytes with brought out nuclei (n), cytoplasm (c) and a well distinct hepatic laminae. (H & E × 400)

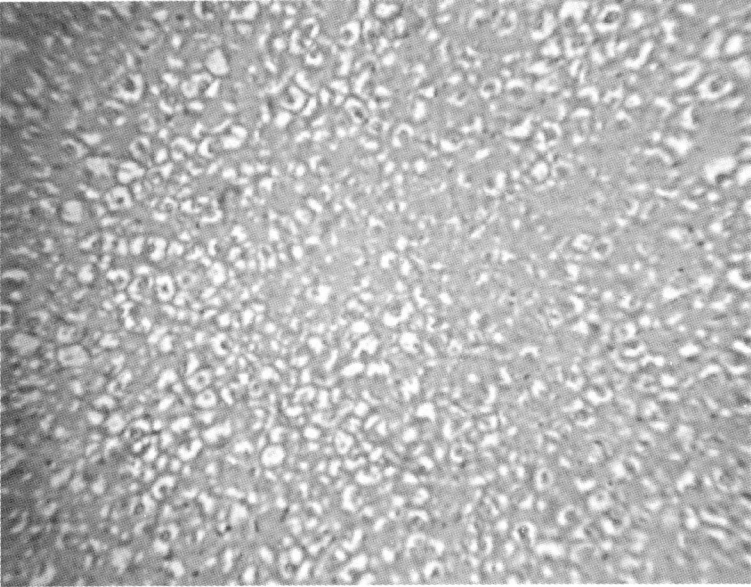

Fig. 12.3. Aceclofenac treated rat (intermediate dose): LM section showing loss of normal architecture and nonzonal macrovesicular lipid accumulation (H & E × 100)

Group IV (high)

Microscopically liver from rats of high dose group showed congestion of sinusoidal spaces, hydropic degeneration with granular eosinophilic cytoplasm of hepatocytes and multiple areas of necrosis. The

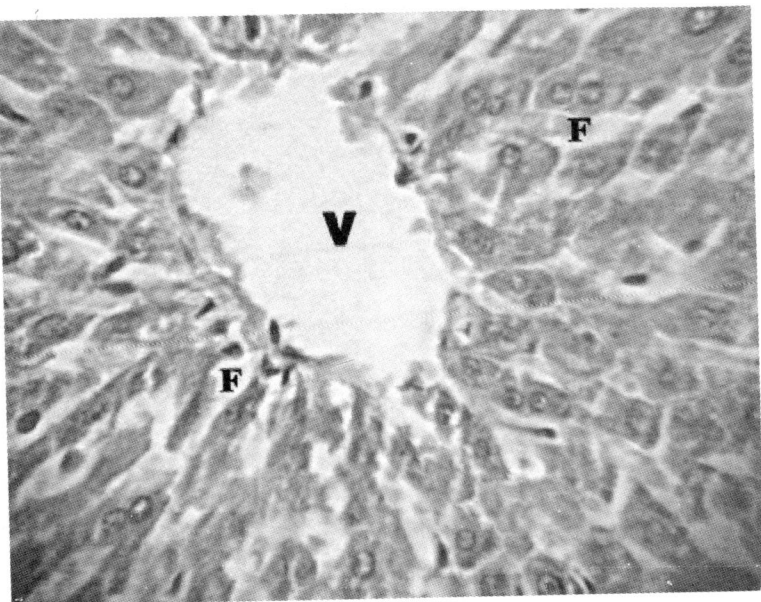

Fig. 12.4. Aceclofenac treated rat (high dose): (i) a central vein (v), (ii) occluded sinusoidal spaces, (iii) hydropic degeneration, (iv) swollen and necrotic hepatocytes, (v) mild fatty degeneration (f). V= extended central vein, F = fatty degradation (H & E × 400)

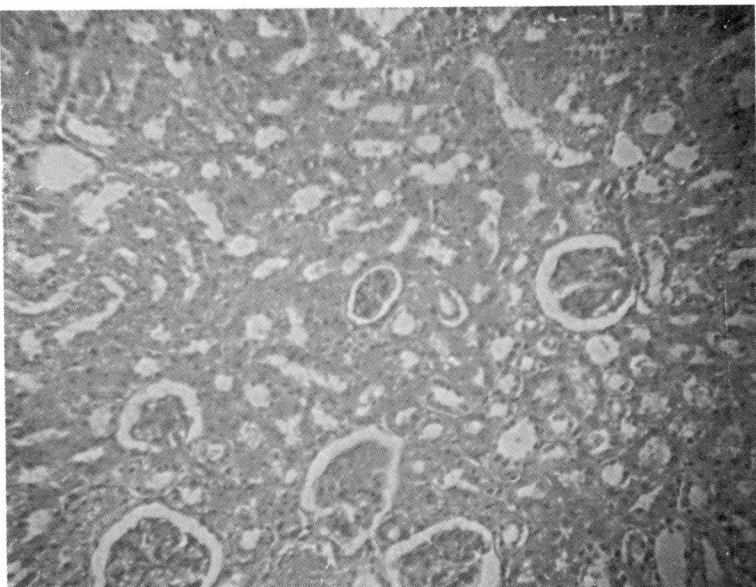

Fig. 12.5. Control rat: Histologic section of rat kidney from the control group. Normal tubular and glomerular structures are seen in the cortex. (Hematoxylin-eosin, × 120)

lesions in kidney microscopically were cystic dilatation of collecting tubules lined by flattened epithelial cells and necrosis of lining epithelium of the kidney tubules. Some renal tubules show (Fig. 12.8) vacuolar degeneration and necrosis of the lining epithelial cells. Kidney tubules also showed retention of urine.

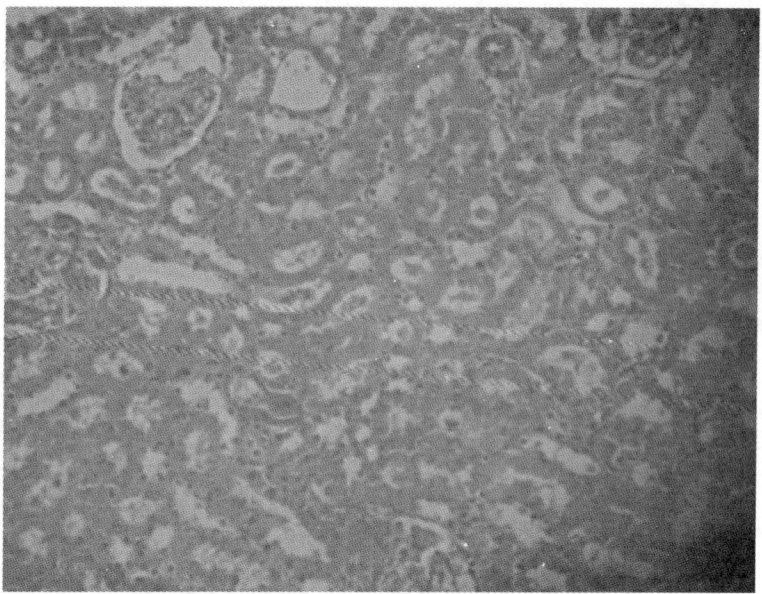

Fig. 12.6. Aceclofenac treated rat (low dose): Histological section of kidney shows almost normal tubular and glomerular structures. (Hematoxylin-eosin, × 120)

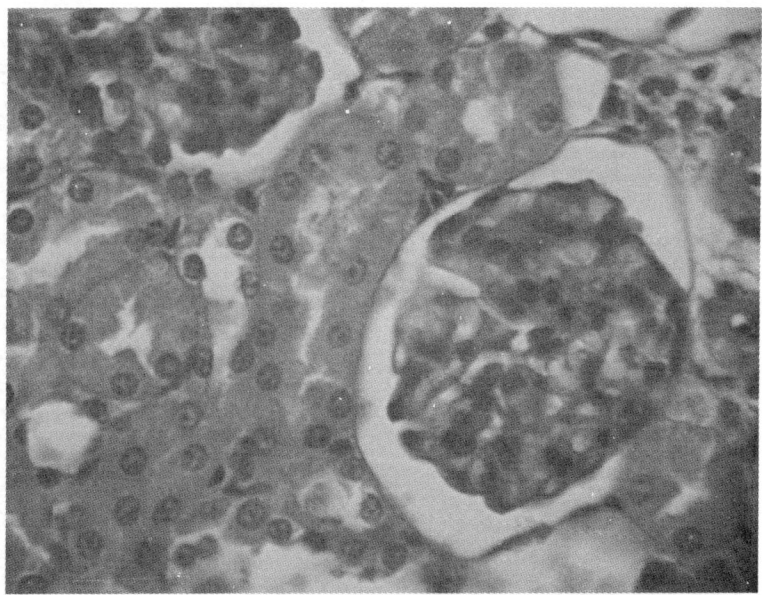

Fig. 12.7. Aceclofenac treated rat (intermediate dose): Histologic examination of rat kidney from intermediate dose treated group showing eosinophilic secretion in the tubulus lumen. (Hematoxylin-eosin, × 400)

Haematological Analysis

The values of RBC, PCV, Hb and neutrophil rates were significantly decreased ($P<0.01$, $P<0.05$, $P<0.05$ and $P<0.01$, respectively) by aceclofenac treatment. WBC count and lymphocyte rates were

PLATE 1

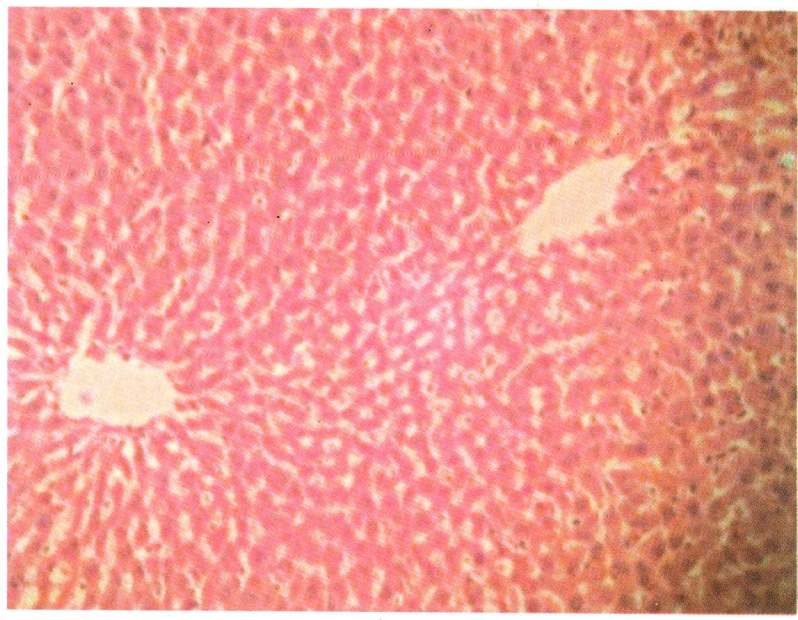

Fig. 12.1. Control rat: LM section of liver showing the normal lobular
histological picture. (H&E×100)

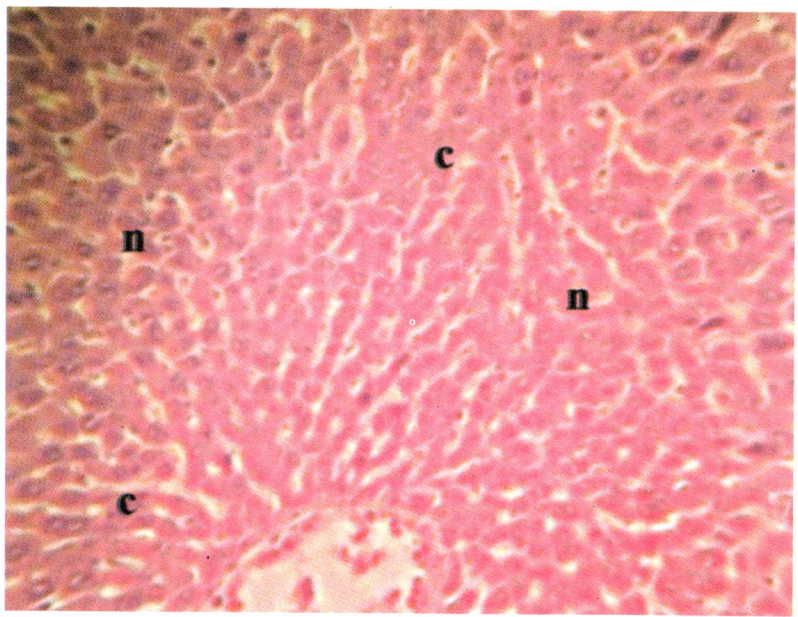

Fig. 12.2. Aceclofenac treated rat (low dose): LM section of liver showing a
normal histological picture. Normal hepatocytes with brought out nuclei (n),
cytoplasm (c) and a well distinct hepatic laminae. (H&E×400)

PLATE 2

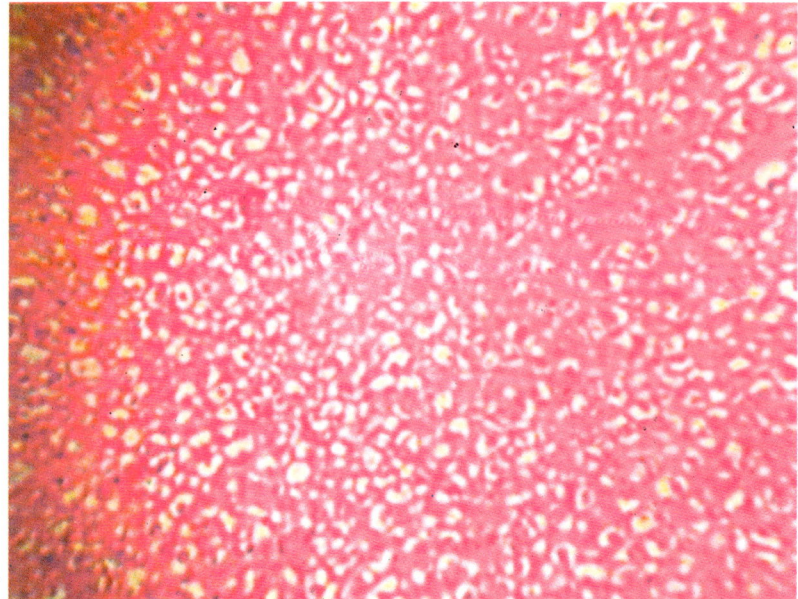

Fig. 12.3. Aceclofenac treated rat (intermediate dose): LM section showing loss of normal architecture and nonzonal macrovesicular lipid accumulation. (H&E×100)

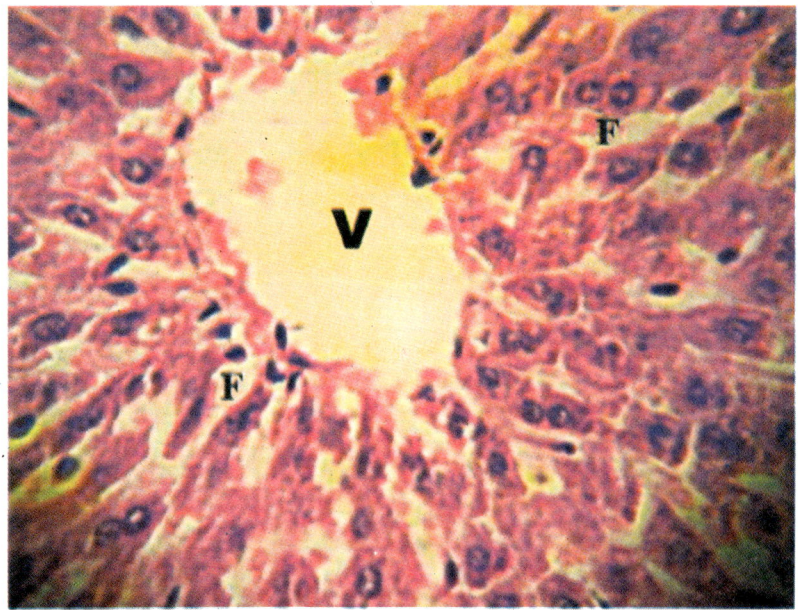

Fig. 12.4. Aceclofenac treated rat (high dose): (i) a central vein (v), (ii) occluded sinusoidal spaces, (iii) hydropic degeneration, (iv) swollen and necrotic hepatocytes, (v) mild fatty degeneration (f). V = extended central vein, F = fatty degradation. (H&E×400)

PLATE 3

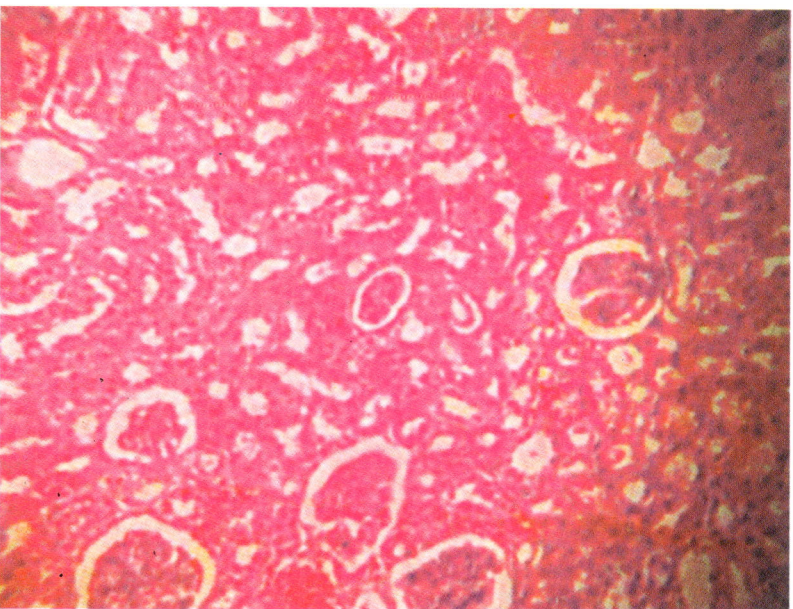

Fig. 12.5. Control rat: Histological section of rat kidney from the control group. Normal tubular and glomerular structures are seen in the cortex. (H&E×120)

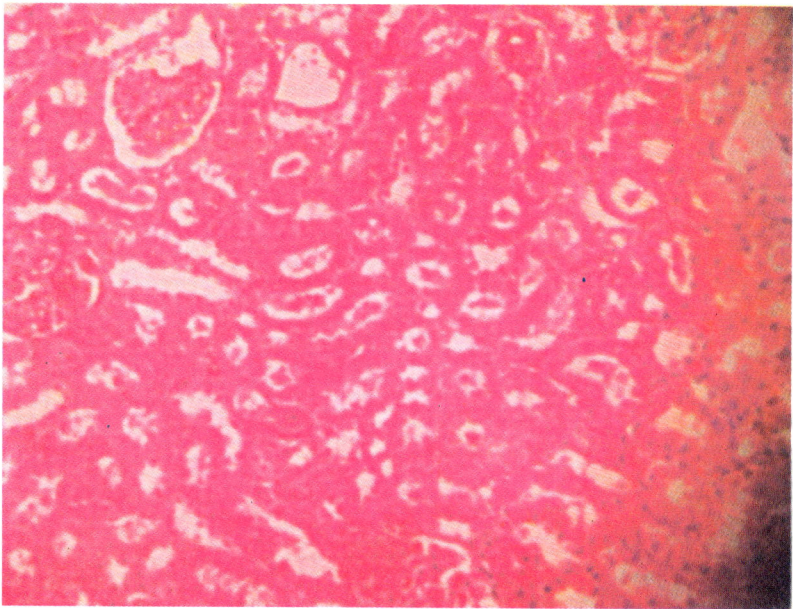

Fig. 12.6. Aceclofenac treated rat (low dose): Histological section of kidney shows almost normal tubular and glomerular structures.
(H&E×120)

PLATE 4

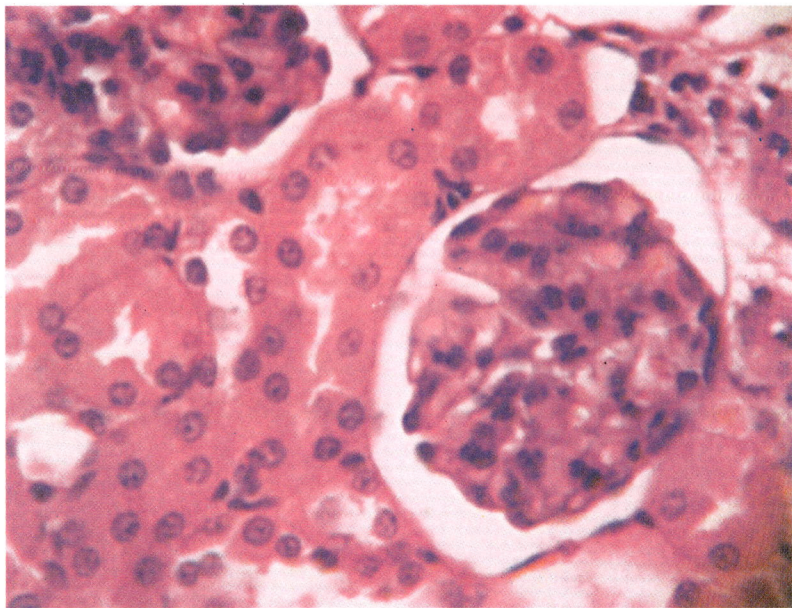

Fig. 12.7. Aceclofenac treated rat (intermediate dose): Histological examination of rat kidney from intermediate dose treated group showing eosinophilic secretion in the tubulus lumen. (H&E×400)

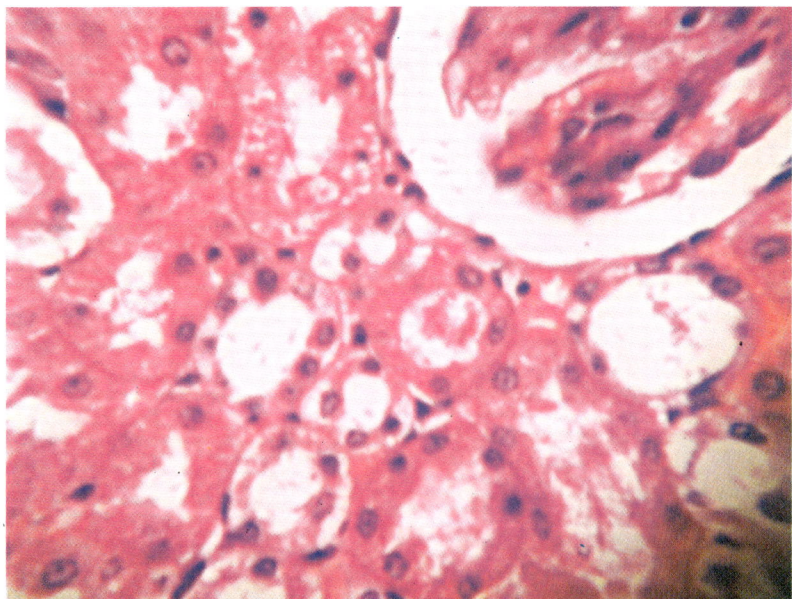

Fig. 12.8. Aceclofenac treated rat (high dose): Histological section of rat kidney from the high dose administered group showing degeneration and epithelial cell necrosis, in the epithelial lining some of the tubules and mononuclear cell infiltration in the interstitium. (H&E×400)

significantly increased (P<0.01 and P<0.01 respectively) by aceclofenac treatment. However, the MCV, MCH, MCHC were not significantly influenced (P>0.05) by aceclofenac.

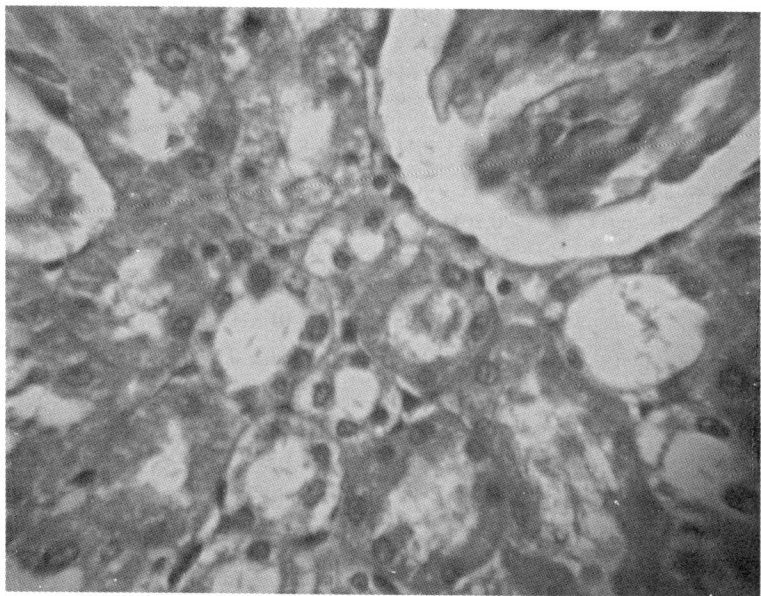

Fig. 12.8. Aceclofenac treated rat (high dose):Histologic section of rat kidney from the high dose administered group showing degeneration and epithelial cell necrosis, in the epithelial lining some of the tubules and mononuclear cell infiltration in the interstitium (Hematoxylin-eosin, × 400)

Table 12.1: Haematological values of male rats in the subchronic study of aceclofenac

Parameter	Control	25 mg/Kg	50 mg/Kg	100 mg/Kg
Red blood cells (×10⁶/mm³)	5.51 ± 0.61	4.33 ± 0.38	4.61 ± 0.85	3.75 ± 0.54
Hemoglobin (g %)	17.22 ± 0.32	18.84 ± 0.26	17.14 ± 0.14	11.27 ± 0.22
Hematocrit (%)	48.91 ± 0.41	48.73 ± 0.28	53.70 ± 0.66	44.28 ± 0.54
Mean corpuscular volume (μm³)	69.44 ± 0.71	43.27 ± 0.28	59.30 ± 0.47	89.10 ± 0.16
Mean corpuscular hemoglobin (pg)	31.51 ± 0.14	29.81 ± 0.32	31.20 ± 0.24	30.21 ± 0.18
Mean corpuscular hemoglobin concentration (%)	35.60 ± 1.34	32.97 ± 0.57	31.04 ± 2.02	33.94 ± 0.68
Platelet (×10⁵/mm³)	5.62 ± 0.98	6.01 ± 1.05	6.59 ± 0.41	4.28 ± 0.89
Total white blood cells (×10³/mm³)	6.41 ± 0.47	5.47 ± 0.69	5.95 ± 1.10	6.98 ± 0.55
Neutrophil (%)	31 ± 2.54	28 ± 1.23	30 ± 0.89	38 ± 1.28
Lymphocyte (%)	61 ± 2.15	74 ± 3.08	77 ± 0.48	74 ± 1.04
Monocyte (%)	01 ± 0.14	02 ± 0.35	01 ± 0.48	01 ± 0.58
Eosinophil (%)	02 ± 0.15	02 ± 0.59	01± 0.78	01 ± 0.33

Values are expressed as mean ± SD. (n=6)

P<0.05, 0.01, 0.001 as compared to respective group

Table 12.2: Haematological values of female rats in the subchronic study of aceclofenac

Parameter	Control	25 mg/Kg	50 mg/Kg	100 mg/Kg
Red blood cells ($\times 10^6/mm^3$)	4.68 ± 0.61	4.21 ± 0.38	4.09 ± 0.85	3.95 ± 0.54
Haemoglobin (g %)	18.43 ± 0.32	18.84 ± 0.26	17.14 ± 0.14	11.27 ± 0.22
Hematocrit (%)	46.53 ± 0.41	48.73 ± 0.28	53.70 ± 0.66	44.28 ± 0.54
Mean corpuscular volume (μm^3)	71.44 ± 0.71	42.67 ± 0.28	61.42 ± 0.47	74.10 ± 0.16
Mean corpuscular hemoglobin (pg)	30.16 ± 0.14	29.81 ± 0.32	31.20 ± 0.24	30.21 ± 0.18
Mean corpuscular hemoglobin concentration (%)	33.60 ± 1.34	32.97 ± 0.57	30.04 ± 2.02	35.94 ± 0.68
Platelet ($\times 10^5/mm^3$)	5.62 ± 0.98	6.01 ± 1.05	6.59 ± 0.41	4.28 ± 0.89
Total white blood cells ($\times 10^3/mm^3$)	5.24 ± 0.47	5.81 ± 0.69	5.95 ± 1.10	6.49 ± 0.55
Neutrophil (%)	39 ± 2.54	28 ± 1.23	33± 0.89	31 ± 1.28
Lymphocyte (%)	90 ± 2.15	74 ± 3.08	77 ± 0.48	62 ± 1.04
Monocyte (%)	01 ± 0.14	02 ± 0.35	02 ± 0.48	01 ± 0.58
Eosinophil (%)	01 ± 0.15	01 ± 0.59	01± 0.78	01 ± 0.33

Values are expressed as mean ± SD. (n=6)

$P < 0.05, 0.01, 0.001$ as compared to respective group

Animals treated with aceclofenac in acute or chronic doses had significantly lower erythrocyte (RBC) count, hemoglobin (Hb) and packed cell volume (PCV) as compared to the controls. The mean cell hemoglobin (MCH) and the mean cell volume (MCV) were significantly greater than controls; while the mean cell hemoglobin concentration (MCHC) was similar in both the groups The erythrocyte diameter was significantly lower whereas the thickness was higher in the treated animals as compared to controls. The total leucocyte (WBC) count, absolute neutrophil count, eosinophil count and lymphocyte count were higher in mice treated with acute or chronic doses of aceclofenac as compared to controls. The monocyte count was higher than the controls in the acutely treated animals while no significant difference was noted in the monocyte counts of sub-chronically treated animals and controls.

Table 12.3: Organ weights relative values (%) of male rats

Organs	Control	25 mg/Kg	50 mg/Kg	100 mg/Kg
Heart	0.3 ± 0.06	0.41 ± 0.03	0.43 ± 0.07	0.45 ± 0.05
Lungs	0.72 ± 0.02	0.89 ± 0.07	0.91 ± 0.09	0.83 ± 0.06
Liver	3.88 ± 0.24	3.75 ± 0.12	3.46 ± 0.16	4.3 ± 0.13
Stomach	1.24 ± 0.14	1.20 ± 0.10	0.98 ± 0.11	1.43 ± 0.9
Kidney	0.63 ± 0.08	0.73 ± 0.03	0.69 ± 0.03	0.89 ± 0.05

Values are expressed as mean ± SD. (n = 6). $P < 0.05, 0.01, 0.001$ as compared to respective group

Biochemical Analysis

The results of the biochemical analysis were depicted in Tables 12.5 and 12.6. It shows the average (n = 6) levels of these biochemical parameters for liver function tests (LFT). A statistical analysis of the

Table 12.4: Organ weights relative values (%) of female rats

Organs	Control	25 mg/Kg	50 mg/Kg	100 mg/Kg
Heart	0.34 ± 0.06	0.46 ± 0.03	0.51 ± 0.07	0.55 ± 0.05
Lungs	0.75 ± 0.02	0.89 ± 0.07	0.93 ± 0.09	0.95 ± 0.06
Liver	3.61 ± 0.24	3.75 ± 0.12	3.89 ± 0.16	4.36 ± 0.13
Stomach	1.43 ± 0.14	1.22 ± 0.10	0.64 ± 0.11	1.67 ± 0.9
Kidney	0.64 ± 0.08	0.75 ± 0.03	0.72 ± 0.03	0.89 ± 0.05

Values are expressed as mean ± SD. (n = 6). P<0.05, 0.01, 0.001 as compared to respective group

results was done as mentioned earlier and was also depicted in the Table. Laboratory analysis of blood samples revealed a significantly elevated levels of serum transaminases and serum bilirubin (total and direct) in the experimental groups (III and IV), (P<0.05) as compared with the control (group I). Elevations in values tend to be relative to the amount of liver damage. From Tables 12.5 and 12.6, it was observed that the level of serum glutamic oxaloacetic transaminase (SGOT) and serum glutamic pyruvic transaminase (SGPT) were significantly higher in the animals fed with high doses of acecolfenac (group-IV), and the levels were seen to be significantly lower in group-I and II animals (P<0.05). The levels of these transaminases were absolutely lower in group I. The total bilirubin and the direct bilirubin levels were significantly higher in the experimental (group III and IV) (P<0.05) when compared with the control and low dose. Biochemical results show serum Alkaline Phosphatase (ALP) and BUN significantly increased in aceclofenac treated group when compared with control. The levels of these transaminases were absolutely lower in group I. The total bilirubin and the direct bilirubin levels were significantly higher in the experimental group III and IV (P<0.05) when compared with the control and group II rats (P<0.05).

Table 12.5: Clinical blood chemistry values of male rats obtained in the subchronic toxicity study of aceclofenac

Parameter	Control	25 mg/Kg	50 mg/Kg	100 mg/Kg
Glucose (mg/dl)	95.14 ± 3.14	92.69 ± 5.12	96.44 ± 2.59	103.08 ± 4.34
BUN (mg %)	22.16 ± 1.26	25.16 ± 2.04	31.57 ± 2.10	41.26 ± 2.42
Total protein (g %)	6.10 ± 0.21	7.04 ± 0.74	5.95 ± 0.48	7.22 ± 0.14
SGOT (IU/L)	230.87 ± 2.44	254.68 ± 4.13	280.89 ± 1.87	312.42 ± 5.04
SGPT (IU/L)	92.34 ± 3.84	99.14 ± 1.94	110.24 ± 2.38	172.52 ± 7.82
ALP (IU/L)	325.77 ± 6.28	342.54 ± 3.50	590.08 ± 4.56	740.45 ± 2.89

BUN – Blood urea nitrogen, SGOT – Serum glutamate oxaloacetic transaminase, SGPT – Serum glutamate pyruvic transaminase, ALP – Alkaline phosphotase

Values are expressed as mean ± SD. (n=6)

P<0.05, 0.01, 0.001 as compared to respective group

Table 12.6: Clinical blood chemistry values of female rats obtained in the subchronic toxicity study of aceclofenac

Parameter	Control	25 mg/Kg	50 mg/Kg	100 mg/Kg
Glucose (mg/dl %)	84.14 ± 3.14	102.69 ± 5.12	99.44 ± 2.59	107.08 ± 4.34
BUN (mg %)	25.16 ± 2.04	22.16 ± 2.04	39.57 ± 2.10	44.26 ± 2.42
Total protein (g %)	6.10 ± 0.21	7 04 ± 0.74	5.95 ± 0.48	7.22 ± 0.14
SGOT (IU/L)	197.87 ± 2.44	206.68 ± 4.13	219.37± 1.87	289.46 ± 5.04
SGPT (IU/L)	82.34 ± 3.84	89.46 ± 1.94	110.24 ± 2.38	157.52 ± 7.82
ALP (IU/L)	310.77 ± 6.28	322.54 ± 3.50	619.08 ± 4.56	684.45 ± 2.89

BUN – Blood urea nitrogen, SGOT – Serum glutamate oxaloacetic transaminase, SGPT – Serum glutamate pyruvic transaminase, ALP – Alkaline phosphotase

Values are expressed as mean ± SD. (n = 6)

$P<0.05, 0.01, 0.001$ as compared to respective group

DISCUSSION

The body weight of high and intermediate dose group was significantly ($P<0.01$) lower than compared to the control group. Low dose group showed normal weight gains and exhibited no such toxic effects.

The RBC, PCV and Hb increased significantly ($P<0.01$) whereas MCV increased significantly ($P<0.01$) in high dose group. The observed fall in hemoglobin concentrations and erythrocyte counts in high dose group might have occurred because of acute loss of blood through faeces (melena). This correlated with the gross pathological change of generalized paleness of all mucous membranes and visceral organs of the body. The observed increase in MCV and decrease in MCHC is suggestive of macrocytic hypochromic anaemia which might have occurred because of acute loss of blood through faeces (melena). High and intermediate dose exerted toxic effect on the liver and the toxic effect on high dose group was more severe compared to that of intermediate dose group, which correlated well with the histopathologic lesions in liver and increase in biochemical parameters ALT and ALP. Aceclofenac at high dose and intermediate dose also has toxic effect on the kidney. The toxic effect in high dose group is more severe compared to that of intermediate dose group, which correlated well with the histopathology of kidney showing severe damage in the high dose group and milder degree of damage in the intermediate dose group and increase in BUN and creatinine concentration in serum.

There was significant ($P<0.01$) increase in organ to body weight ratio in case of liver which may be due to fatty changes in the liver and also due to diarrhoea and dehydration. Similar increase in relative liver weight due to fatty change, diarrhoea and dehydration was observed in broiler chicks fed diet containing ochratoxin A. There was also significant ($P<0.01$) increase in kidney to body weight ratio, which may be due to cystic dilatation and retention of urine in tubules and also due to diarrhea and dehydration. Similar increase in relative kidney weight due to cystic dilatation and retention of urine was observed in newborn rats with partial unilateral ureteric obstruction. Thus, from the present study, it was concluded that aceclofenac at high and intermediate dose is hepatotoxic and nephrotoxic in rats.

REFERENCES

1. Aithal GP, Day CP. (2007) Nonsteroidal anti-inflammatory drug-induced hepatotoxicity. Clin Liver Dis. 11(3): 563–575.

2. Manov I, Motanis H, Frumin I, Iancu TC. (2006) Hepatotoxicity of anti-inflammatory and analgesic drugs: ultrastructural aspects. Acta Pharmacol Sin. 27, 259–272.

3. Hussaini SH, Farrington EA. (2007) Idiosyncratic drug – induced liver injury: an overview. Expert opinion on drug safety. 6: 673–684.

4. Vane, J.R. (1971) Inhibition of prostaglandin synthesis as a mechanism for aspirin like drugs. Nature New Biol. 231: 232–235.

5. Vane, J.R., Bakhle, Y.S. and R.M.Botting. (1998) Cyclooxygenases 1 and 2. Annu. Rev. Pharmacol. Toxicol. 38: 97–120.

6. Dubols, R.N., Abramson, S.B., Gofford, L., Gupta, R.A., Slmon, L.S., VanDe Putte, L.B. and Lipsky, P.E. (1998) Cyclooxygenase in biology and disease. FASEB J. 12: 1063–1073.

7. Brogden, R.N., Wiseman, L.R., (1996) Aceclofenac: A review of its pharmacodynamic properties and therapeutic potential in the treatment of rheumatic disorders and in pain management. Drugs. 52: 113–124.

8. Hawkey, C.J. (1990) Non-steroidal anti-inflammatory drugs and peptic ulcers. Facts and figures multiply, but do they add up? BMJ. 300: 278–284.

9. Retiman, S., Frankel, A.S., (1957) A Colorimetric method for the determination of serum glutamic oxaloacetic and glutay pyruvic transaminases. Am. J. Clin. Pathol. 28: 53–56.

10. King, J. (1965) The hydrolases-acid and alkaline phosphatase, Practical Clinical Enzymology, Van, D (ed), (Nostrand company Ltd., London) pp. 191–208.

11. Malloy, H.T. (1937) The determination of bilirubin with the photoelectric colorimeter. J. Bio.Chem. 119: 481–485.

12. Lowry, O.H., Rosebrough, N.J., Farr, A.L. and Randall, R.J.1951 Protein measurement with folin phenol reagent. J. Bio. Chem. 193: 265–275.

13. Galighar, A. E., Kozloff, E. N. (1971) Essentials of practical microtechnique. 2nd edn, vol. 210, Lea and Febigu, Philadelphia, pp.77.

14. Armitage, P., and Berry, G., (1985) In Statistical methods in medical research, 2nd edn. London. Blackwell scientific publications. 201–203.

Protocol for Bioequivalence Study

BIOEQUIVALENCE OF TABLET/CAPSULES

Protocol No.

RATIONALE

This study is required to assess the bioequivalence **Tablet/Capsules**

Aims and Objectives

The aim and objective of the present study is to evaluate the pharmacokinetic parameters and to compare the single dose oral bioavailabiliity of Tablet (TEST preparation) of **Company Address** with **Tablet** (REFERENCE preparation) of **Company Name.** The study will be carried out, by utilizing a typical two-period, randomized, two-way complete crossover design in 12 healthy male, human volunteers.

ETHICAL REVIEW AND CONSENT PROCEDURE

Ethics Review Procedure

Guidelines as drawn up by the Institutional Review Board will be followed with regard to the treatment of human volunteers in the study. These guidelines meet the requirements of the US Code of Federal Regulations (Title 21, Part 56), the Declarations of Helsinki and the Canadian MRC Guidelines. The protocol and the informed consent form will be submitted to the Ethical Committee prior to the initiation of the study. The approval of the Ethical Committee will be taken in advance of the study commencement. The study will not proceed until the approval of the Ethical Committee has been received.

Informed Consent

Before recruitment and enrollment into the study, each prospective candidate will be given a full explanation of the study. Once this essential information is provided to the subject and once the physician in charge has the conviction that he understands the implications of participating in the study, the subject will be asked to sign the informed consent form.

STUDY DESIGN

The bioequivalence of the TEST preparation will be assessed utilizing a typical two-period, randomized, two-way complete crossover design in 12 healthy, male, human volunteers. There will be 2 dosing sessions with a washout period of 7 days between the two sessions. All the volunteers are required to participate in two dosing sessions. In each dosing session, volunteers received either of the TEST or REFERENCE preparation of Tablet as a single dose, only on the study day, as per the randomization code at a fixed time.

Volunteers will be given code numbers by the bio-statistician of the CPU (Clinical Pharmacology Unit). They will be allocated to the treatment A / B (Reference or Test preparation) in accordance with the randomization code. Neither the personnel in charge of the determination of plasma levels nor the physician and nursing staff in charge of the clinical aspects, in particular of the adverse reactions, is informed of the sequence of administration. The volunteer is not totally blinded in that he aware that he is receiving different formulations of a same drug without being informed of which formulation is Test or Reference. The investigator preparing the drugs for administration is the only person who knows the code.

SUBJECT SELECTION CRITERIA

Adult, healthy, male, human volunteers with 18 to 40 years of age will be selected from the panel of volunteers recruited by CPU. The selected volunteers will be screened for inclusion in the study within 21 days before the commencement of the study.

Screening Tests

The screening examination will include complete physical and clinical examination, various biochemical and hematological tests. They are:

1. Complete physical and Clinical examination including personal and family history.
2. Complete hemogram
3. LFT (Liver Function Tests) S. Bilirubin, S. Proteins, SGOT, SGPT, Alk. Phosphatase
4. RFT (Renal Function Tests): BUN, S. Creatinine
5. S. Proteins
6. Blood Sugar (Fasting)
7. Virological Tests: HIV Antibody, HBS Ag.
8. Routine Urine Examination

Inclusion Criteria

(a) The minimum and maximum ages for participating in this study will be respectively 18 and 40 years of age.
(b) Only males will be eligible for the study.
(c) Subjects will be within 15% of their ideal weight as of Life Insurance Company's table.
(d) Healthy (eligible after physical, clinical, hematological and biochemical examination)
(e) Normal ECG
(f) Normal blood pressure and heart rate as measured after resting supine for three minutes. Normal BP is taken to be 100 to 150 mm Hg systolic and 50 to 90 mm Hg diastolic supine. Normal heart rate is taken to be 50 to 90 beats per minute.
(g) The volunteer should be able to communicate well with the investigator.
(h) Availability of subject for the entire study period and willingness to adhere to protocol requirements as evidence by written informed consent.
(i) To be a non-smoker.

Exclusion Criteria

    (a) History of hypersensitivity to the study drug or related products.

    (b) Significant history or presence of gastrointestinal, liver or kidney disease, or any other conditions known to interfere with the adsorption, distribution, metabolism or excretion of common medications.

    (c) Significant history of asthma, chronic bronchitis or other bronchospastic condition.

    (d) Significant history or presence of glaucoma, cardiovascular or haematological disease.

    (e) Any clinically significant illness during the 4 weeks prior to day 1 of this study.

    (f) Maintenance therapy with any drug, or history of drug dependence, alcohol abuse, or serious neurological or psychological disease.

    (g) Participation in a clinical trial with an investigation drug within 30 days prior to day 1 of this study.

    (h) Use of any systemic medication (including OTC preparations) within 14 days preceding day 1 of this study.

    (i) HIV and Australian antigen positive subjects.

    (j) Clinically relevant abnormal physical and/or clinical findings at the screening.

    (k) Abnormal ECG

    (1) Loss of greater than 400 ml of blood, in the period 0 to 12 weeks before entry to the study or during the study.

    (m) Serious adverse reaction or hypersensitivity to any drug.

    (n) Inability to communicate or cooperate with the investigator due to language problem, poor mental development or impaired cerebral function.

Subject Withdrawal

The study team will make every reasonable effort to complete the study. If a subject wishes to leave the study at any time, he will be permitted to do so. Every reasonable effort will be made to complete a final assessment.

    A subject may withdraw from the study in any of the following circumstances:

1. Serious adverse events
2. Major violation of the protocol
3. Withdrawal of the consent
4. Termination of the study by the sponsor
5. Any systemic illness occurring during the study period requiring intake of other drugs

    Any subject discontinuing the trial medication prematurely because of reasons 1 or 5 will be replaced.

PRODUCT INFORMATION

Reference Preparation (A):

Tablet
Mfg. by

Test Preparation (B):

Tablet
Mfg. by

DOSING PATTERN

The volunteers will be randomized on the previous day of study day 1. In study session I, each volunteer will receive either the TEST preparation of Tablet or the REFERENCE preparation of Tablet as single dose on the study day at a fixed time. In study session II, this order will be reversed as per the randomization. For the purpose of accurate sampling time for all samples, study medications will be administered at intervals of 1 minute to groups of 2 subjects. Study medication will be given with 240 ml water at room temperature.

CONCOMITANT MEDICATION

Subjects will be informed well in advance not to take any drug for at least 14 days prior to the study. They will be specifically reminded that this includes cold preparations, vitamins and antacid preparations. In addition, no concomitant medication will be permitted during the study period. Each subject will be specifically questioned on these points prior to drug administration. If a subject admits drug ingestion, the Principal Investigators will decide whether the subject will be permitted to remain in the study depending on the drug used. The drug and dose will be noted and reported in the case report form. The volunteers will also be instructed to refrain from consuming alcohol, smoking or any other stimulant drinks, during this period.

SUPPLY OF DRUGS

The TEST drug in suitable packing and appropriate condition, along with the Certificate of Analysis and the statement of expiry date will be supplied by the sponsor to the clinical pharmacologist at least 7 working days prior to the study date. The TEST drug will be stored under the control of the clinical pharmacologist in locked cupboard at ambient temperature unless otherwise advised by the sponsor. Prior to the commencement of the study, the sponsor will supply a complete Test Material Data Sheet (TMDS) indicating the Test material identity, purity, stability, appearance, handling and safety instructions. The TMDS may be cross-reference to the sponsor's certificate of analysis.

DRUG ACCOUNTABILITY

Drug Inventory Records will be maintained by the Principal Investigator. The Principal Investigator will maintain an inventory record of the drug received and dispensed. Medication will be provided to study subjects only. Upon completion or termination of the study, unused drug will be returned to the Sponsor in their original containers. This includes containers of drug, which are partially used as well as unopened supplies, which are never dispensed. A retained sample of study supplies may be until at least 1 year following receipt of marketing approval by the sponsor, at which time the samples will be destroyed or returned when directed in writing by the sponsor.

BLOOD COLLECTION

All the volunteers will assemble at 6.00 a.m. on the study day 1 of each session, after overnight fasting of at least 10 hrs. Their TPR, BP will be recorded and an indwelling intravenous cannula will be introduced with strict aseptic precautions in the anticubital vein for blood collection.

They will receive either of the study preparations (Reference/Test) according to their code nos. with 240 ml of water. The exact clock time will be calculated according to the drug administration schedule. The first blood sample (T = 0) will be collected immediately prior to drug administration. The clock time of all blood draws will be recorded and reported for each subject. Any deviation from the sampling schedule will be recorded in the subject's sampling time sheet.

Sampling time sheets for all subjects will be attached in the final report. A total of 14 blood samples will be collected from anticubital vein at 0 hr. (before drug administration) 0.5, 1.0, 1.5, 2.0, 3.0, 4.0, 6.0, 8.0, 10.0, 12.0, 18.0, 24.0 and 48.0 hrs in coded, centrifuge tubes containing EDTA. Blood samples will be centrifuged immediately, the plasma separated into duplicate polypropylene tubes and stored frozen at $-100°$ C. The tubes will be labeled with volunteer code number, sampling time and study date. This code will not reveal formulation identity.

DIETARY CONTROL

A standardized breakfast, lunch and dinner will be served to subjects at 3, 6–8 and 14 hours respectively after drug ingestion. Water will be provided *ad libitum* until 1.0 hour predose. Fluid intake will be controlled and consistent for the first 3.0 hours following drug administration as follows: drug will be given 240 ml of water at room temperature and no fluids except one cup of non-caffeine-containing soft drink will be allowed till 3 hours postdose. On the study day volunteers will be permitted normal activities, excluding strenuous exercise.

ANALYSIS OF BLOOD SAMPLES

The concentration of blood samples will be analyzed by HPLC/GC with ECD method developed and validated in the Analytical Laboratory. The analytical method will be validated prior to the start of study.

ADVERSE EVENTS

Abnormal symptoms/signs will be monitored, during the study period and for one week after the study period and if noticed, their details will be entered in the case report sheets and tabulated at the end of the study.

EMERGENCY PROCEDURES

Emergency equipment and drugs will be available in the CPU. In the unlikely event that they are required their use will be documented. Copies of randomization schedule will be held by the biostatistician in sealed envelopes. The clinical pharmacologist may request that the envelope be opened in the event of emergency.

CRITICAL PHASES

Medical and nursing personnel will supervise all critical phases of the study. Any deviations from the protocol will be recorded. The clinical pharmacologist will personally monitor all the events.

CONDITIONS FOR MODIFYING OR TERMINATING THE STUDY PROTOCOL AMENDMENTS

All changes or revisions of this protocol will be documented, signed and dated by the Chief Investigator. The reason for the amendment will be stated.

CONFIDENTIALITY

It is agreed that the information contained in this protocol and the results of the study will not be disclosed to others, without written authorization from the sponsor except to staff involved in the study.

DOCUMENTATION

Data Entry

All data obtained during the course of the clinical phase of the study will be recorded directly and legibly into the Case Record Form in black ink. The clinical pharmacologist will prepare the case record forms.

Data Protection

When personal data on subjects are stored or processed by computer the date must be protected to prevent their disclosure to unauthorized third parties.

EVALUATION OF PHARMACOKINETIC PARAMETERS

The plasma levels produced by the administration of the studied drug in each volunteer and corrected for the measured content of the dosage form will be used to establish the pharmacokinetic profile of TEST and REFERENCE preparations. The plasma drug level profile will be presented in tabular and graphical forms. The following pharmacokinetic parameters of TEST and REFERENCE preparations will be calculated for each subject.

- C_{max} (Peak plasma concentration)
- t_{max} (Time to maximum plasma concentration)
- $AUC_{(0.24)}$ (The area under plasma concentration time curve 0 to 24 hours)
- $AUC_{(0-\alpha)}$ (The area under plasma concentration time curve 0 to α)
- $t_{1/2}$ (Elimination half life)
- K_{el} (Elimination rate constant)

C_{max} and t_{max} are observed values. K_{el} is the elimination rate constant estimated by a linear least-squares regression analysis of the individual concentrations observed as a function of time during the elimination phase. The elimination $t_{1/2}$ is obtained using the following relationship:

$$t_{1/2} = \frac{0.693}{K_{el}}$$

STATISTICAL ANALYSIS

Usual descriptive analysis including the mean and standard deviation (SD) will be used for variables such as the height, weight and age. These statistical parameters including coefficient of variance will also be used to describe plasma concentrations at each individual time point as well as the pharmacokinetic parameters. Following statistical test will be applied on untransformed (t_{max}, C_{max}, $AUC_{(0-t)}$, $AUC_{(0-\alpha)}$) and log-transformed pharmacokinetic data (C_{max}, $AUC_{(0-t)}$, $AUC_{(0-\alpha)}$).

1. Anova of t_{max}, C_{max}, $AUC_{(0-t)}$, $AUC_{(0-\alpha)}$ will be subjected to a 3-way Anova accounting for subjects, period and treatment.

2. 90% confidence interval (CI) consistent with two one-sided t-test with the significance level of 5% for untransformed and log-transformed parameters (t_{max}. C_{max}, $AUC_{(0-t)}$, $AUC_{(0-\alpha)}$).

Products will be considered to be bioequivalent, if the 90% confidence interval (CI) of difference in the average values of logarithmic AUC and C_{max} between TEST and REFERENCE preparations is within the acceptable range of Log (0.8) to Log (1.25).

QUALITY ASSURANCE: GOOD LABORATORY PRACTICE AND GOOD CLINICAL PRACTICE

Studies will be conducted in accordance with guidance and good clinical research practice in the European Community approved by the CPMP in July 1990.

REPORTING OF TEST RESULTS

The report will include:

1. Samples

1. Brand name and lot No. of the reference product. Code No. or name, lot No. and lot size of test product
2. Type of dosage form
3. Name of drug substances
4. Labeled contents or potencies

2. Results of Tests

1. Summary
2. Bioequivalence studies

Following will be described:
(a) Experimental conditions
  (i) **Subjects**
    Age, sex, body weight and other data obtained by laboratory tests will be described.
  (ii) **Drug administration**
  (iii) Fasting time, co-administered water volume, and times of drug administration and food ingestion are described along with the menu and content of meal and times of food ingestion during studies.
  (iv) **Assay**
    Procedure and summary of validation.
(b) Results
  (i) Individual subject data: It includes tables showing drug levels in biological fluids at each sampling time, C_{max}, AUC_{0-t}, $AUC_{0-\alpha}$, K_{el} and t_{max}. The correlation coefficient for determining K_{el} will be reported together with time points used. The ratios of C_{max} and AUC_{0-t} of test product to those of reference product in each individual will be reported. Figures comparing individual drug level-time profiles of the two products drawn on a linear scale are illustrated.
  (ii) Average and standard deviations: Tables showing averages and standard deviations of raw data of drug levels in biological fluids at each time point, C_{max}, AUC_{0-t}, $AUC_{0-\alpha}$, K_{el} and

t_{max}, and the ratios of average of C_{max} and AUC_{0-t}, of test product to those of reference product will be reported. Figures comparing average drug level-time profiles of the two products drawn on a linear scale are described.

(iii) Statistical analysis and equivalence assessment: It includes the analysis of variance tables for C_{max}, AUC_{0-t}, $AUC_{0-\alpha}$, K_{el} and t_{max}, which are logarithmically transformed when required. The 90% confidence interval for C_{max} and AUC0-t or alternative statistical results will be reported. For other parameters, statistical testing results of the null-hypotheses will be reported where the average values of test and reference products are assumed to be equivalent.

(iv) Others: Information on dropouts (data, reasons), monitoring records of health of subjects.

After completion of the study a draft report will be prepared and sent to the sponsor. Upon receipt of approval or amendments or 4 weeks from the date of issue of the draft report, the final report will be sent.

BIOEQUIVALENCE/BIOAVAILABILITY STUDY VOLUNTEER CONSENT FORM

1. I understand that the investigation will involve the administration of .... the undersigned voluntarily agree to take part in the study: titled as: Bioequivalence of .... X .... on .... study days in .... dosing sessions at the interval of .... days.

2. I have been given a full explanation by the member of the study team, of the nature, purpose and likely duration of the study and what I will be expected to do and I have been advised about my discomfort and possible ill-effects on my health or well-being which he believes may result.

3. I have been given the opportunity to question the study team, on aspects of the study and have understood the advise and information given as a result.

4. I agree to comply with any instruction given during the study and to cooperate faithfully with the study team, and to tell immediately, if I suffer from any deterioration of any kind in my health or well being or any unexpected or unusual symptoms, however, they may have arisen.

5. I agree that I will not seek to restrict the use to which the results of the study may be put in particular, I accept that they may be disclosed to regulatory authorities for medicines.

6. I understand that I am free to withdraw from the study at any time without needing to justify my decision.

Signature of the Volunteer: Address: ....
....
Date: ....

Signature of the Investigator

Date:

Protocol for Clinical Trial

CLINICAL TRIAL TO ASSESS EFFICACY AND SAFETY OF CEFPIROME AND SULBACTAM IN BACTEREMIA/SEPTICEMIA AND SEVERE INFECTIONS IN INTENSIVE CARE PATIENTS

TABLE OF CONTENTS

I. INTRODUCTION

Cefpirome is a fourth generation cephalosporin. In comparison with second, third and other fourth generation derivatives it has higher activity against gram-positive pathogens, good activity against *Pseudomonas aeruginosa* and a markedly improved stability to the chromosomal class I cephalosporinase commonly produced by enterobacter spp.. It has been shown to be effective in the treatment of bacteremia in a number of trials.

Sulbactam is a derivative of basic penicillin nucleus. It is a irreversible inhibitor of beta-lactamase produced by resistant bacteria.

Cefpirome and sulbactam is a synergistic antimicrobial combination with a marked in vitro antibacterial activity against a broad spectrum of organisms.

The combination of cefpirome/sulbactam has potential to improve cost-effectiveness of antimicrobial therapy as they replace regimens that use multiple antibiotics or antibiotics with relatively high incidence of adverse reactions. In cefpirome/sulbactam combination, sulbactam improves cefpirome's activity against beta-lactamase producing strains.

Based on this rationale, Venus Remedies has developed a fixed dose combination cefpirome 2 G with sulbactam 1 G for treatment of bacteremia/septicemia.

II. OBJECTIVES

The objective of the study is to assess the efficacy and safety of Cefpirome and Sulbactam FDC in patients of bacteraemia/septicemia.

III. STUDY DESIGN

A. Design: Multicenter, open label, non-comparative study

B. Phase of the trial: Phase III

C. Duration: 3 months

D. Number of patients: 100 (25 in each centre X 4 centres)

IV. STUDY TREATMENT AND ADMINISTRATION

A. Dosing Schedule

The combination will be given in a dose of 1.5 to 3.0 grams twice daily. Detailed instruction will be provided with the sample for proper dosage and administration.

B. Study Drugs Control and Administration

At the commencement of the study the investigator will issue the drug as per the dosage requirement of the patients to the clinical research assistant (CRA) and the empty vial of the same will be collected next day in exchange of the stock for the next day and so on till completion of the study.

The investigator will, at his/her discretion, discontinue the drug for patients whose sensitivity reports, when organisms cultured, are resistant to the drug being given to the patient and the new drug prescribed will be recorded and the patient will be taken off the protocol and counted as ineligible for ITT and PP analysis. However, the details of the organism and its sensitivity will be recorded and analysed as explained later.

The CRA will maintain a separate drug account for each patient in the drug record book.

V. STUDY POPULATION AND SUBJECT ELIGIBILITY SUBJECT SELECTION

The study group will include hospitalized patients suffering from bacteremia/septicemia proven or suspected to be caused or complicated by gram-negative organisms. The patient will be eligible to participate if the liver and kidney functions are normal (or in case of dysfunction up to 2 times the normal value) and he agrees to be a part of the study and gives an informed consent. Subjects must be above the age of 18 years (age of consent) and must not have received either of the antibiotic in previous 4 weeks, and must be capable of giving informed consent. Specific inclusion and exclusion criteria will be described.

VI. CONDUCT OF STUDY

After informed consent is obtained, patients will receive the medication for 7–10 days (provided the sensitivity report obtained justifies such use as mentioned above).

When 7 days of treatment are over and if in the opinion of the attending doctor an oral antibiotic is necessary, the same may be prescribed and recorded on the CRF.

The patients will be observed for any side effects during treatment, hypersensitivity reaction, headache, insomnia, abdominal cramps, diarrhea, nausea and urinary retention.

Study Parameters: Efficacy

Clinical improvement and bacteriological conversion (when applicable) are the primary endpoints and are defined as a subject who is

- resolution of primary symptoms
- sensitivity tests show absence of infecting organisms detected on initial culture on completion of 7 days of treatment and again 7 days after discontinuation of injectable antibacterial treatment.

Secondary endpoints

- time for complete resolution defined as
- complete resolution of all symptoms of urinary tract infection
- the number of days after beginning treatment with FDC to discharge.

Tolerability

Tolerability of the FDC is to be determined by the number and severity of adverse effects reported spontaneously (defined as those reported by subject or his/her attendant/relative) and also the adverse effect observed by the attending medical or nursing staff.

VII. ADVERSE EVENTS

A. Adverse Events Monitoring

Any adverse effect observed, regardless of the treatment group or suspected causal relationship to the study drug, will be recorded on the adverse event page of the case record form. Events involving adverse drug reaction, with details of onset and further events during the study will be recorded.

Follow-up of the adverse event even after the date of discontinuation of the therapy is required if the adverse event or its sequel persists. Follow-up is required until the event or its sequel resolves or stabilizes at a level acceptable to the investigator and to clinical monitor. For all adverse events, the attending investigator must pursue and obtain information adequate to determine the outcome of the adverse event and must opine whether the adverse reaction could have occurred due to the treatment administered.

B. Withdrawal from Study

A withdrawal occurs when the enrolled patient ceases participation in the study, regardless of the circumstances, prior to the completion of the protocol. Typically subjects may withdraw from the study for the following reasons:

1. At the request of the subject;

2. The investigator considers that a subject's health will be compromised due to an adverse experience, or concomitant illness that develops after entering the study;

3. The subject is recognized after entry to be uncooperative, or a consistent violator of protocol requirements.

4. For any subject who withdraws from the study before the study is completed, the investigator will:

   - Complete the case report form, indicating the date of and explanation of the early withdrawal from the study. If possible, provide an overall evaluation of safety of the assigned treatment;

   - Arrange for alternate medical care of the discontinued subject if necessary.

   - and record on appropriate case report form pages any follow-up of subjects discontinued for adverse experiences.

A withdrawal must be reported immediately to the clinical monitor if it is due to a serious adverse event. The investigator will record the reason for withdrawal from the study, provide or arrange for appropriate follow-up (if required) for such patients, and document the course of the patient's condition.

VIII. ETHICAL CONSIDERATION

A. Ethics Committee Review and Communication

Ethics committee approval will be obtained from an independent ethics committee (National Ethics Committee) before initiating the trial.

It will be the responsibility of the ethics committee to review and accord its approval to a trial protocol to safeguard right, safety, and well-being of all trial subjects.

B. Informed Consent

Prior to the enrollment into the study, informed consent will be obtained from each subject, in accordance with the standard operating procedures. The investigator will explain the patients the objectives of the trial and will ask them to sign the Informed Consent Form after having understood its contents completely.

While taking the informed consent the patients will be informed of their possibility of experiencing some side effects. Patient will also be informed that he/she is free to withdraw from the study any time without giving any reason.

C. Subject Confidentiality, Including Ownership of Data and Coding Procedure

The confidentiality of the identification of all participating patients will be maintained. Security and confidentiality of study data will be assured.

IX. STUDY MONITORING AND SUPERVISION

A. Monitoring of Study

A representative of the sponsor will visit or communicate with the investigator at regular intervals so as to assess the progress of the study and the adherence to the protocol. The investigator should maintain source documents such as consultation reports, complete history and examinations, etc. for possible review by sponsor and/or drug authorities. The investigator will permit the representative to review all the source documents.

B. Recording of Data

The investigator will ensure that all data are entered promptly and accurately, in accordance with specific instructions accompanying the case report forms supplied by the sponsor. An explanation for the omission of any required data should appear on the appropriate page.

The signature of the investigator or his/her appropriate designee will appear on each page of the case report form.

C. Clinical Supplies

The sponsor will provide the investigator with adequate quantities of the following materials to permit completion of the study:

1. Protocol
2. Case record forms and informed consent form
3. Drug samples

The investigator should maintain adequate records of the receipt and disposal of all study drugs supplied. Any unused medication will be returned to the sponsor at the conclusion of the study. The investigator should ensure that the study medication is stored in a limited access area and protected from extremes of light, temperature and humidity.

D. Time Schedule

The total duration of the trial will be 3–4 months, i.e. the study should be finished and available data of the patients should be sent for statistical analysis by the monitor.

E. Secrecy Agreement

The results and the data obtained from the above study will be property of Venus Remedies and under no circumstances will either a part or the entire study be published, presented or discussed with others without obtaining a prior written permission from Venus Remedies.

X. STATISTICAL ANALYSIS

Categorical data between the baseline and post treatment values will be compared with the χ^2 test, and continuous data will be compared with *Student's t-test.*

Data on the number of cases that need to be taken off protocol because the bacteria are reported to be resistant to the study drug, will help in determining the appropriateness or otherwise of the FDC drug to be given as a routine empirical therapy before bacteriological reports in such serious infections.

APPENDIX I OF PROTOCOL

Serious Adverse Events Form

1. Patient Details:

   Patient name: ....

   Patient initials: ....

   Gender: ....

   Age: ....

   Weight: ....

   Height: ....

2. Suspected Drugs

   (a) Generic name of the drug: ....

   (b) Indications for which the drug was prescribed or tested: ....

   ....

   (c) Dosage form and strength:

   ....

   (d) Daily dose and regimen:

   ....

   (e) Route of administration:

   ....

   (f) Starting date and time of the day: ..../ ...... / .... at ....

   (g) Stopping date and time: .... / ...... / .... at ....

   (h) Duration of treatment:

   ....

3. Other Treatments Details

   ....

   ....

   ....

   ....

4. Details of Suspected Adverse Drug Reaction

   (a) Description of reaction:

   ....

   ....

   ....

   (b) Start date and time of onset of reaction: ..../....../............. at ....

   (c) Stop date and time of onset of reaction: ..../....../............. at ....

   (d) Duration of reaction: ....

   (e) Dechallenge and/or rechallenge: ....

   ....

   ....

(f) Hospital setting:

....

5. Outcome
   (a) Information on recovery and any sequelae:

   ....

   ....

   (b) Results of specific tests and/or treatment that may have been used:

   ....

   ....

   ....

   (c) Possible relationship to the suspected reaction:

   ....

   ....

   ....

   (d) Any relevant information to facilitate assessment:

6. Details about the Investigator
   (a) Name: ....
   (b) Address: ....

   ....

   ....

   (c) Telephone numbers: ....
   (d) Specialty: ....
   (e) Date of reporting the event to licensing authority: ..../........./............
   (f) Date of reporting the event to ethics committee: ..../........./.............

   (g) Signature of investigator: ....

APPENDIX II OF PROTOCOL

Informed Consent Form

Study Title : Clinical Trial to assess efficacy and safety of
Cefpirome and Sulbactam in Bacteremia/Septicemia
and severe infections in Intensive Care Patients

Study Number:

Subject's Name: .... Subject's Initials: ....

(i) I confirm that I have read and understood the information sheet dated for the above study and have had the opportunity to ask questions.

(ii) I understand that my participation in the study is voluntary and that I am free to withdraw at any time, without giving any reason, without my medical care or legal rights being affected.

(iii) I understand that the sponsor of the clinical trials, others working on the sponsor's behalf, the ethics committee and the regulatory authorities will not need my permission to look at my health records, both in respect of current study and any further research that may be conducted in relation to it, even if I withdraw from the trial. I agree to this access. However, I understand that my identity will not be revealed in any information released to third parties or published.

(iv) I agree not to restrict the use of any data or results that arise from this study provided such a use is only for scientific purpose.

(v) I agree to take part in the above study.

.... Date: ..../........../............

Signature (or thumb impression) of the
subject/legally acceptable representative:

Signatory's name: ....

Signature of the investigator .... Date: ..../........../............

Name of the investigator ....

Signature of the witness: .... Date: ..../........../............

Name of the witness: ....

Appendix 2

MULTICENTRIC, OPEN-LABEL, NON-RANDOMIZED CLINICAL TRIAL TO ASSESS EFFICACY AND SAFETY OF THE FIXED-DOSE COMBINATION OF CEFPIROME AND SULBACTAM IN BACTEREMIA/SEPTICEMIA AND SEVERE INFECTIONS IN INTENSIVE CARE PATIENTS

PRINCIPAL INVESTIGATOR:

STUDY INITIATION:

STUDY COMPLETION:

SPONSOR: ....
....
....

SYNOPSIS

Short title/study phase	To assess efficacy and safety of the fixed-dose combination of Cefpirome and Sulbactam in Bacteremia/Septicemia and severe infections in Intensive Care Patients Phase III
Indication	Bacteremia/Septicemia and severe infections in Intensive Care Patients

Manufacturer of investigational product and address	(Name and address of the company)
Investigational product, dosage and route of administration	Fixed-dose combination of Cefpirome and Sulbactam, Parenteral, 1.5 to 3.0 grams twice daily.
Reference product, dosage and route of a dministration	Since this is an open-label study, there is no reference drug
Primary objective	To assess the efficacy of Cefpirome and Sulbactam FDC in Bacteremia/Septicemia and severe infections in Intensive Care Patients
Secondary objective	To assess the efficacy of Cefpirome and Sulbactam FDC in Bacteremia/Septicemia and severe infections in Intensive Care Patients
Measurement procedures for objectives (endpoints)	Primary parameters Clinical improvement and bacteriological conversion (when applicable) are the primary endpoints and are defined as a subject who is <ul><li>Afebrile for 48 hours with resolution of symptoms</li><li>Sensitivity tests show absence of infecting organisms detected on initial culture on completion of 7 days of treatment and again 7 days after discontinuation of injectable antibacterial treatment</li></ul>
Patient profile (most important inclusion criteria)	Hospitalized patients suffering from Bacteremia/Septicemia and severe infections
Short title/study phase	To assess efficacy and safety of the fixed-dose combination of Cefpirome and Sulbactam in Bacteremia/Septicemia and severe infections in Intensive Care Patients Phase III Proven or suspected to be caused or complicated by gram-negative organisms.
Duration of treatment	7–10 days
Study design	Multicentric, open label, non-comparative study control
Adverse events identification	Events involving adverse drug reaction, with details of onset and further events during the study, will be recorded.
Number of study centres and countries	Centre 1. (Doctor's Name)
Overall number of patients, minimum and maximum number per center (if possible)	27 patients
Planned start of recruitment Planned end of treatment Planned end of follow-up (if applicable)	
Plan for data analysis	

DISCUSSION AND OVERALL CONCLUSION

The main finding of this multicentric study was that Cefpirome with Sulbactam was effective as conventional broad-spectrum antimicrobial combinations for treatment of bacteremia and septicemia. For all infections combined, the clinical cure rate at the end of therapy was as high as 82%.

All the clinically evaluable population had an isolated pathogen that was identified before treatment began. Cefpirome-Sulbactam combination eradicated 94% of all pathogens. Accordingly, this study extends the findings of previously published clinical studies, which found Cefpirome to be effective for the treatment of complicated lower respiratory tract and urinary tract infections.

This study also demonstrated that Cefpirome-Sulbactam has an excellent safety and tolerability profile with adverse events primarily limited to injection site reactions, e.g. Phlebitis, and effects on the gastrointestinal tract, e.g. Diarrhea, nausea. None of the adverse events were related to the drug therapy.

Innumerous trials have established that *E. coli* and *P. aeruginosa* as the prime organisms causing uncomplicated and complicated UTI. Similarly, gram-positive organisms like Strepto. Pneumoniae and Staph. Aureus have been attributed to respiratory tract infections as well as skin and soft tissue infections. Less than half of theses isolates obtained from hospitalized patients with UTIs are susceptible to broat-spectrum penicillins; *in vitro* resistance rates are also high against both old and new fluoroquinolones. Cefpirome monotherapy is found to be effective clinically and bacteriologically effective in the management of hospitalized patients with complicated infections. A recent surveillance study, conducted in Latin America among hospitalized patients with complicated infections, found that Cefpirome had excellent *in vitro* susceptibility against many antibiotic-resistant gram-positive and gram-negative isolates (91.7%). However, the ESBL (Extended Spectrum Beta Lactam) bacteria have mastered the art of hydrolyzing even fourth generation cephalosporins. Because antimicrobial resistance among uropathogens causing community-acquired UTIs (e.g. *E. coli)* is increasing, especially against ampicillin and trimethoprim-sulfamethoxazole (TMP-SMX), new antibiotic options are needed to treat these infections. The present combination of Cefpirome and Sulbactam realizes clinical cure of 100%. The data from our trial are promising; it appears that Cefpirome monotherapy is an effective empiric agent for the treatment of potentially antibiotic-resistant uropathogens and serious UTIs.

Few clinical studies describe the "real-world" approach to treatment of serious infections with empiric antimicrobial therapy. Limitations of this study included the nonblinded design and the low number of patients in UTI. Although these limitations necessitate careful interpretation, evaluation of clinical success at the end of therapy reflects "real-world" clinical practice and is noteworthy.

In summary, the relatively recent availability of potent broad-spectrum antimicrobial agents has decreased the need for combination antimicrobial therapy for the treatment of hospitalized patients with serious infections. This study enrolled "real-world" hospitalized patients with complicated bacteremia and septicemia. Empiric use of Cefpirome-Sulbactam resulted in high rates of clinical success and bacteriologic eradication.

Overall, Cefpirome-Sulbactam combination is an effective and well tolerated in the treatment of bacteremia and septicemia.

If they are to prescribe appropriate empiric therapy, physicians must be knowledgeable about geographic differences in the causes and susceptibility patterns of organisms associated with serious community-acquired infections. Use of inappropriate empiric antimicrobial therapy may lead to increased rates of mortality and morbidity. As with any serious infection, antimicrobial therapy should be tailored when culture and susceptibility data become available.

GUIDELINES FOR TOXICITY STUDY

Protocol

Introduction

It is essential to use at least two species (usually a rodent and a non-rodent) in the evaluation of the potential toxicity of a drug because species differ in their responses to toxic agents. It is also unwise to use a homogenous strain (inbred strain) in toxicity test, and the aim should be to discover new and unexpected effects of a drug in animals of wider variability like random bred animals. A drug effect that is seen both in the rat and in the dog probably involves a common physiologic mechanism that is likely to be present in the humans, whereas an effect seen only in one of the two species indicates that the same is peculiar to that species, and is less likely to be present in the 3rd species. For instance, a toxic effect observed only in rats or dogs would indicate its probability of occurring in about 25 per cent in cases of man; while an effect observed in both rats and dogs would indicate a probability of 80 per cent.

Table 1: OECD Organization of Economic Cooperation and Development guidelines for acute, subchronic and chronic oral and dermal toxicity studies are:

Test	*Tide*
Acute	Acute Oral Toxicity
	Acute Dermal Toxicity
	Acute Oral Toxicity — Fixed Dose Method
	Acute Oral Toxicity — Acute Toxic Class Method
	Acute Oral Toxicity — Up and Down Procedure
Subchronic	Repeated Dose 28 Day Oral Toxicity Study in Rodents
	Repeated Dose 90 Day Oral Toxicity Study in Rodents
	Repeated Dose 90 Day Oral Toxicity Study in Non-rodents
	Repeated Dose Dermal Toxicity: 21/28-day Study
	Subchronic Dermal Toxicity: 90-day Study
Chronic	Chronic Toxicity Study
	Combined Chronic Toxicity/Carcinogenicity Study

ACUTE TOXICITY STUDIES

Acute toxicity is the toxicity produced by a pharmaceutical when it is administered in one or more doses during a period not exceeding 24 hours. Acute toxicity studies in animals are usually necessary for any pharmaceutical intended for human use. The information obtained from these studies is useful in choosing doses for repeat-dose studies, providing preliminary identification of target organs of toxicity, and, occasionally, revealing delayed toxicity. Acute toxicity studies may also aid in the selection of starting doses for Phase I human study, and provide information relevant to acute overdosing in humans.

SUBACUTE AND SUBCHRONIC TOXICITY STUDIES

Subacute and subchronic toxicity determines the systemic effect of repeated doses of materials or their extracts for not less than 24 hours and not greater than 10% of the total lifespan of the test animal. The test substance or extract is administered to the animal for 14 days, and is observed each day for signs of toxicity, i.e. weight change, appetite, signs of disease or abnormal behavior. Then, the effects are evaluated and a histopathology is conducted on all animals.

Purpose

The purpose of this document is to suggest the format for final reports (right column) and to provide instructions for the creation of PDF Version 1.3 electronic submission documents (left column). Regarding PDF, both "bookmarks" and "links" are referenced. Bookmarks and links are similar in function in that both provide the reader with a way to move efficiently through a document as well as across documents. Bookmarks are a type of link that appear in the navigation pane on the left side of the PDF reader user screen. Links appear within the body of a document as blue text. They permit the reader to jump to other locations with related information in the same document or other electronic documents.

The same format is appropriate for **oral, dermal, primary eye irritation,** and **skin irritation** studies. Slightly different formats are appropriate for **acute toxicity-inhalation** and **skin sensitization** study reports.

Table 2: Acute Oral and Dermal; Primary Eye Irritation and Skin Irritation Studies

Instructions to Create PDF	*Document Format*
Create bookmarks for each item in the document format column.	• Study Title Page, • Statement of Data confidentiality. No confidentiality claims can be made for electronically submitted studies at this time, • GLP Statement, • QA Statement.
Create bookmarks for each item in table of contents.	• Table of Contents.
Create links in summary to related text and tables in body of study report or appendices.	• Executive Summary, Summary of Materials and Methods, Summary of Results, • Test Material Identification, • Test Animal Identification, • Test Material Administration.
Create links to related text, tables, or appendices.	• Results, Mortality, Clinical Observations, Gross Necropsy, • Body Weights, • Deviations, • Tables.

How are LD/LC50 Tests Done?

In nearly all cases, LD50 tests are performed using a pure form of the chemical. Mixtures are rarely studied.

The chemical may be given to the animals by mouth (oral); by applying on the skin (dermal); by injection at sites such as the blood veins (iv- intravenous), muscles (im - intramuscular) or into the abdominal cavity (ip - intraperitoneal).

Table 3: Acute inhalation toxicity studies

Instructions to Create PDF	*Document Format*
Create bookmarks for each item in the Document format column.	• Study Title Page, • Statement of Data Confidentiality. No confidentiality claims can be made for electronically submitted studies at this time, • GLP Statement, • QA Statement.
Create bookmarks for each item in table of contents.	• Table of Contents.
Create links in summary to related text and tables in body of study report or appendices.	• Executive Summary, Summary of Materials and Methods, Summary of Results, • Test Material Identification, • Test Animal Identification, • Method, Ambient Conditions, Exposure Description (Chamber/Period), Atmospheric Generation Model, Chamber Concentration Measurements, Particle Size Evaluation.
Create links to related text, tables, or appendices.	• Results Mortality, Exposure Concentration, MMAD/GSD, Clinical Observations, Gross Necropsy, • Body Weights, • Deviations, • Tables.

The LD50 value obtained at the end of the experiment is identified as the LD50 (oral), LD50 (skin), LD50 (i.v.), etc. as appropriate. Researchers can do the test with any animal species but they use rats or mice most often. Other species include dogs, hamsters, cats, guinea-pigs, rabbits, and monkeys. In each case, the LD50 value is expressed as the weight of chemical administered per kilogram body weight of the animal and it states the test animal used and route of exposure or administration; e.g. LD50 (oral, rat)—5 mg/kg, LD50 (skin, rabbit)—5 g/kg. So, the example "LD50 (oral, rat)—5mg/kg" means that 5 mg of that chemical for every 1 kg body weight of the rat, when administered in one dose by mouth, causes the death of 50% of the test group.

If the lethal effects from breathing a compound are to be tested, the chemical (usually a gas or vapour) is first mixed in a known concentration in a special air chamber where the test animals will be placed. This concentration is usually quoted as parts per million (ppm) or milligrams per cubic metre (mg/m). In these experiments, the concentration that kills 50% of the animals is called an LC50 (Lethal Concentration 50) rather than an LD50. When an LC50 value is reported, it should also state the kind of test animal studied and the duration of the exposure, e.g. LC50 (rat) — 1000 ppm/4 hr or LC50 (mouse) — 5 mg/m^3/ 2hr.

ED50 and LC50

The dose of a drug that is pharmacologically effective for 50% of the population exposed to the drug or a 50% response in a biological system that is exposed to the drug.

LC50: (Lethal Concentration 50) is the concentration of a chemical which kills 50% of a sample population. This measure is generally used when exposure to a chemical is through the animal breathing it in, while the LD50 is the measure generally used when exposure is by swallowing, through skin contact, or by injection.

REPEATED DOSE 28-DAY ORAL TOXICITY STUDY IN RODENTS; PRINCIPLE OF THE TEST

The test substance is orally administered daily in graduated doses to several groups of experimental animals, one dose level per group for a period of 28 days. During the period of administration the animals are observed closely, each day for signs of toxicity. Animals which die or are killed during the test period are necropsied and at the conclusion of the test surviving animals are killed and necropsied. A 28-day study provides information on the effects of repeated oral exposure and can indicate the need for further longer term studies. It can also provide information on the selection of concentrations for longer term studies. The data derived from using the TG should allow for the characterization of the test substance toxicity, for an indication of the dose response relationship and the determination of the No-Observed Adverse Effect Level (NOAEL).

DESCRIPTION OF THE METHOD

Selection of Animal Species

The preferred rodent species is the rat, although other rodent species may be used. If the parameters specified within this TG 407 are investigated in another rodent species a detailed justification should be given. Although it is biologically plausible that other species should respond to toxicants in a similar manner to the smaller species may result in increased variability consequent to technical challenges of dissecting smaller organs. In the international validation program for the detection of endocrine disrupture, the rat was the only species used. Commonly used laboratory strains of young healthy adult animals should be employed. Females should be nulliparous and non-pregnant. Dosing should begin as soon as possible after weaning, and, in any case, before the animals are nine weeks old. At the commencement of the study the weight variation of animals used should be minimal and not exceed 20% of the mean weight of each sex. When a repeated oral dose is conducted as a preliminary to a longer-term study, preferably animals from the same strain and source should be used in both studies.

Housing and Feeding

The temperature in the experimental animal room should be 22 °C, the relative humidity should be at least 30% and preferably not to exceed 70% other than during room cleaning, the aim should be 50–60%. Lighting should be artificial, the sequence being 12 hours light, 12 hours dark. For feeding, conventional laboratory diets may be used with an unlimited supply of drinking water. The choice of diet may be influenced by the need to ensure a suitable admixture of a test substance when administered by this method. Animals may be housed individually, or be caged in small groups of the same sex; % or group caging, not more than five animals should be housed per cage. The feed should be regularly analysed for contaminants. A sample of the diet should be retained until finalisation of the report.

Preparation of Animals

Healthy young adult animals are randomly assigned to the control and treatment groups. Cages should be arranged in such a way that possible effects due to cage placement are minimized. The animals are identified uniquely and kept in their cages for at least five days prior to the start of the study to allow for acclimatisation to the laboratory conditions.

Preparation of Doses

The test compound is administered by gavage or via the diet or drinking water. The method of oral administration is dependent on the purpose of the study, and the physical/chemical properties of the test material. Where necessary, the test substance is dissolved or suspended in a suitable vehicle. It is recommended that, wherever possible, the use of an aqueous solution/suspension be considered first, followed by consideration of a solution/emulsion in oil (e.g. corn oil) and then by possible solution in other vehicles. For vehicles other than water the toxic characteristics of the vehicle must be known. The stability of the test substance in the vehicle should be determined.

PROCEDURE

Number and sex of animals at least 10 animals (five female and five male) should be used at each dose level. If interm kills are planned, the number should be increased by the number of animals scheduled to be killed before the completion of the study. Consideration should be given to an additional satellite group of ten animals (five per sex) in the control and in the top dose group for observation of reversibility, persistence, or delayed occurrence of toxic effects, for at least 14 days post-treatment.

Dosage

Generally, at least three test groups and a control group should be used, but if from assessment of other data, no effects would be expected at a dose of 1000 mg/kg body weight/day, a limit test may be performed. If there are no suitable data available, a range finding study may be performed to aid the determination of the doses to be used. Except for treatment with the test substance, animals in the control group should be handled in an identical manner to the test group subjects. If a vehicle is used in administering the test substance, the control group should receive the vehicle in the highest volume used. O Dose levels should be selected taking into account any existing toxicity and (toxico-) kinetic data available for the test compound or related materials. The highest dose level should be chosen with the aim of inducing toxic effects but not death or severe suffering. Thereafter, a descending sequence of dose levels should be selected with a view to demonstrating any dosage related response and no-observed-adverse effects at the lowest dose level (NOAEL). Two to four-fold intervals are frequently optimal for setting the descending dose levels and addition of a fourth test group is often preferable to using very large intervals (e.g. more than a factor of 10) between dosages. In the presence of observed general toxicity (e.g. reduced body weight, liver enlargement, heart or lung effects, etc.) observed effects on immune, neurological or endocrine sensitive endpoints should be interpreted with caution.

Limit Test

If a test at one dose level of at least 1000 mg/kg body weight/day or, for dietary or drinking water administration, an equivalent percentage in the diet, or drinking water (based upon body weight determinations), using the procedures described for this study, produces no observable toxic effects and if toxicity would not be expected based upon data from structurally related compounds, then a full study using three dose levels may not be considered necessary. The limit test applies except when human exposure indicates the need for a higher dose level to be used.

Administration of Doses

The animals are dosed with test substance daily 7 days each week for a period of 28 days. When the test substance is administered by gavage, this should be done in a single dose to the animals using a stomach tube or a suitable intubation cannula. The maximum volume of liquid that can be administered at one time depends on the size of the test animal. The volume should not exceed 1 ml/100g body weight except in the case of aqueous solutions where 2 ml/100 g body weight may be used. Except for irritating or corrosive substances, which will normally reveal exacerbated effects with higher concentrations, variability in test volume should be minimized by adjusting the concentration to ensure a constant volume at all dose levels. For substances administered via the diet or drinking water it is important to ensure that the quantities of the test substance involved do not interfere with normal nutrition or water balance. When the test substance is administered in the diet either a constant dietary concentration (ppm) or a constant dose level in terms of the animals' body weight may be used; the alternative used must be specified. For a substance administered by gavage, the dose should be given at similar times each day, and adjusted as necessary to maintain a constant dose level in terms of animal body weight. Where a repeated dose study is used as a preliminary to a long term study, a similar diet should be used in both studies.

Observations

The observation period should be 28 days. Animals in a satellite group scheduled for follow-up observations should be kept for at least 14 days without treatment to detect delayed occurrence, or persistence of, or recovery from toxic effects. General clinical observations should be made at least once a day, preferably at the same time(s) each day and considering the peak period of anticipated effects after dosing. The health condition of the animals should be recorded, at least twice daily, all animals are observed for morbidity and mortality. Once before the first exposure (to allow for within-subject comparisons), and at least once a week thereafter, detailed clinical observations should be made in all animals. These observations should be made outside the home cage in a standard arena and preferably at the same time, each time. They should be carefully recorded, preferably using scoring systems, explicitly defined by the testing laboratory. Effort should be made to ensure that variations in the test conditions are minimal and that observations are preferably conducted by observers unaware of the treatment. Signs noted should include, but not be limited to, changes in skin, fur, eyes, mucous membranes, occurrence of secretions and excretions and autonomic activity, e.g. lacrimation, piloerection, pupil size, unusual respiratory pattern. Changes in gait, posture and response to handling as well as the presence of clonic or tonic movements, stereotypies (e.g. excessive grooming, repetitive circling) or bizarre behaviour (e.g. self-mutilation, walking backwards) should also be recorded. In the fourth exposure week sensory reactivity to stimuli of different types (e.g. auditory, visual and proprioceptive stimuli) assessment of grip strength and motor activity assessment should be conducted. Further details of the procedures that could be followed are given in the respective references. However, alternative procedures than those referenced could be used. Functional observations conducted in the fourth exposure week may be omitted when the study is conducted as a preliminary study to a subsequent subchronic (90-day) study. In that case, the functional observations should be included in this follow-up study. On the other hand, the availability of data on functional observations from the repeated dose study may enhance the ability to select dose levels for a subsequent subchronic study. Exceptionally, functional observations may also be omitted for groups that otherwise reveal signs of toxicity to an extent that would significantly interfere with the functional test performance. During the last four days before necropsy, the oestrus cycle of all females could be determined (optional) by taking vaginal smears starting on day 25 at the latest. These observations will provide information regarding the stage of ovarian cycle at the time of sacrifice and assist in histological evaluation of estrogen sensitive tissues.

Body Weight and Food/Water Consumption

All animals should be weighed at least once a week except in the case of studies where dose is administered by gavage when weights should be recorded at least every second day and preferably daily to allow accurate calculation of daily dose. Measurements of food consumption should be made at least weekly. If the test substance is administered via the drinking water, water consumption should also be measured at least weekly.

Haematology

The following haematological examinations should be made at the end of the test period: haematocrit, haemoglobin concentration, erythrocyte count, reticulocytes, Heinz bodies, total and differential leucocyte count, platelet count and a measure of blood clotting time/potential. Blood samples should be taken from a named site just prior to or as part of the procedure for killing the animals, and stored under appropriate conditions. Animals should be fasted prior to killing.

Clinical Biochemistry

Clinical biochemistry determinations to investigate major toxic effects in tissues and, specifically, effects on kidney and liver, should be performed on blood samples obtained from all animals just prior to or as part of the procedure for killing of the animals (apart from those found moribund and/or intercurrently killed). Investigations of plasma or serum shall include sodium, potassium, glucose, total cholesterol, urea, creatinine, total protein and albumin, at least two enzymes indicative of hepatocellular effects (such as alanin aminotransferase, aspartate aminotransferase, alkaline phosphatase, y-glutamyl trans-peptidase and glutamate dehydrogenase), and bile acids. Measurements of additional enzymes (of hepatic or other origin) and bilirubin may provide useful information under certain circumstances. Optionally, the following urinalysis determinations could be performed during the last week of the study using timed urine volume collection; appearance, volume, osmolality or specific gravity, pH, protein, glucose and blood/blood cells. In addition, studies to investigate plasma or serum markers of general tissue damage should be considered. Other determinations that should be carried out, if the known properties of the test substance may, or are suspected to, affect related metabolic profiles include calcium, phosphate, triglycerides, specific hormones, methaemoglobin, and cholinesterase. These need to be identified for chemicals in certain classes or on a case-by-case basis. Although in the international evaluation of the endocrine related endpoints a clear advantage for the determination of thyroid hormones (T_3, T_4) and TSH could not be demonstrated, it may be helpful to retain plasma or semi samples to measure T_3, T_4 and TSH (optional) if there is an indication for an effect on the pituitary-thyroid axis. These samples may be frozen at $-20°$ for storage. The following factors may influence the variability and the absolute concentrations of the hormone determinations:

- time of sacrifice because of diurnal variation of hormone concentrations
- method of sacrifice to avoid undue stress to the animals that may affect hormone concentrations
- test kits for hormone determinations that may differ by their standard curves.

Definitive identification of thyroid-active chemicals is more reliable by histopathological analysis rather than hormone levels. Plasma samples specifically intended for hormone determination should be obtained at a comparable time of the day. It is recommended that consideration should be given to T_3, T_4 and TSH determinations triggered based upon alterations of thyroid histopathology. The numerical values obtained when analysing hormone concentrations differ with various commercial assay kits. Consequently, it may not be possible to provide performance criteria based upon uniform historical data. Alternatively, laboratories should strive to keep control coefficients of variation below 25 for T_3 and T_4 and below 35 for TSH. All concentrations are to be recorded in ng/ml. If historical baseline data are inadequate, consideration should be given to determination of haematological and clinical biochemistry variables before dosing commences or in a set of animals not included in the experimental groups.

PATHOLOGY GROSS NECROPSY

All animals in the study shall be subjected to a full, detailed gross necropsy which includes careful examination of the external surface of the body, all orifices, and the cranial, thoracic and abdominal cavities and their contents. The liver, kidneys, adrenals, testes, epididymides, prostate + seminal vesicle with coagulating glands as a whole, thymus, spleen, brain and heart of all animals (apart from those found moribund and/or intercurrently killed) should be trimmed of any adherent tissue, as appropriate, and their wet weight taken as soon as possible after dissection to avoid drying. Care must be exercised when trimming the prostate complex to avoid puncture of the fluid-filled seminal vesicles. Alternatively, seminal vesicles and prostate may be trimmed and weighed after fixation. In addition, the wet weight could be determined for paired ovaries and uterus (optional) as soon as possible after dissection, to avoid drying. The thyroid weight (optional) could be determined after fixation. Trimming should also be done very carefully and only after fixation to avoid tissue damage. Tissue damage could compromise histopathology analysis. The following tissues should be preserved in the most appropriate fixation medium for both the type of tissue and the intended subsequent histopathological examination: all gross lesions, brain (representative regions including cerebrum, cerebellum and pons), spinal cord, eye, stomach, small and large intestines (including Peyer's patches), liver, kidneys, adrenals, spleen, heart, thymus, thyroid, trachea and lungs (preserved by inflation with fixative and then immersion), gonads (testis and ovaries), accessory sex organs (uterus, epididymides, prostate + seminal vesicle with coagulating glands), vagina, urinary bladder, lymph nodes (preferably one lymph node covering the route of administration and another one beside this proximal draining node), peripheral nerve (sciatic or tibial) preferably in close proximity to the muscle, skeletal muscle and bone, with bone marrow (section or, alternatively, a fresh mounted bone marrow aspirate). It is recommended that testes be fixed by immersion in Bouin's or modified Davidson's fixative after poking several holes in the tunica albuginea at the both ends of the organ with a needle to permit fixative penetration. The clinical and other findings may suggest the need to examine additional tissues. Also any organs considered likely to be target organs based on the known properties of the test substance should be preserved. The following tissues may give valuable indication for endocrine-related effects: Gonads (ovaries and testes), accessory sex organs (uterus, cervix, vagina, epididymides, seminal vesicles with coagulation gland, dorsolateral and ventral prostate), pituitary, male mammary gland, and adrenal gland. Changes in male mammary gland have not been sufficiently documented but this parameters may be very sensitive to substances with estrogenic action. Observation of organs/tissues that are not listed in paragraph 33 is optional. In the international test program some evidence was obtained that subtle endocrine effects by chemicals with a low potency for affecting sex hormone homeostasis may be identified by disturbance of the synchronisation of the oestrus cycle in different tissues and not so much by frank histopathological alterations in female sex organs. Although no definitive proof was obtained for such effects, it is recommended that specific emphasis should be given by histopathology on synchronisation of cyclic alterations in ovaries (follicular, thecal, and granulosa cells), uterus, cervix, vagina, and pituitary in comparison to the stage of cycle as determined by vaginal smears.

Histopathology

Full histopathology should be carried out on the preserved organs and tissues of all animals in the control and high dose groups. These examinations should be extended to animals of all other dosage groups, if treatment-related changes are observed in the high dose group. All gross lesions shall be examined. When a satellite group is used, histopathology should be performed on tissues and organs identified as showing effects in the treated groups.

DATA AND REPORTING DATA

Individual data should be provided. Additionally, all data should be summarised in tabular form showing for each test group the number of animals at the start of the test, the number of animals found dead during the test or killed for humane reasons and the time of any death or humane kill, the number showing signs of toxicity, a description of the signs of toxicity observed, including time of onset, duration, and severity of any toxic effects, the number of animals showing lesions, the type of lesions, their severity and the percentage of animals displaying each type of lesion. When possible, numerical results should be evaluated by an appropriate and generally acceptable statistical method. The statistical methods should be selected during the design of the study. For quality control it is proposed that historical control data are collected and that for numerical data coefficients of variation are calculated, especially for the updated parameters. These data can be used for comparison purposes when actual studies are evaluated.

Test Report

The test report must include the following information: 1. Test substance: - physical nature, purity and physicochemical properties; - identification data. 2. Vehicle (if appropriate): - justification for choice of vehicle, if other than water. 3. Test animals: - species/strain used; - number, age and sex of animals; - source, housing conditions, diet, etc.; - individual weights of animals at the start of the test - justification for species if not rat.

Test report

The test report must include the following information:

Test substance:

– physical nature, purity and, where relevant, physicochemical properties (including isomerisation); – identification data, including CAS number.

Vehicle (if appropriate):

– justification for choice of vehicle, if other than water.

Test animals:

– species/strain used-microbiological status of the animals, when known-number, age and sex of animals (including, where appropriate, a rationale for use of males instead of females);
– source, housing conditions, diet, etc.

Test conditions:

– rationale for initial dose level selection, dose progression factor and for follow-up dose levels;
– details of test substance formulation including details of the physical form of the material administered;
– details of the administration of the test substance including dosing volumes and time of dosing;
– details of food and water quality (including diet type/source, water source).

Results:

– body weight/body weight changes;
– tabulation of response data and dose level for each animal i.e. animals showing signs of toxicity including nature, severity, duration of effects, and mortality;

- individual weights of animals at the day of dosing, in weekly intervals thereafter, and at the time of death or sacrifice;
- time course of onset of signs of toxicity and whether these were reversible for each animal;
- necropsy findings and any histopathological findings for each animal, if available;
- LD50 data;
- statistical treatment of results (description of computer routine used and spreadsheet tabulation of calculations).

Discussion and interpretation of results.

Index

Author Index

Subject Index

Reader's Notes